To Shirley; (handwritten)

W9-BHX-923

SOBER
for the *health* of it

A NUTRITIONAL APPROACH TO THE TREATMENT OF ALCOHOLISM

Peace & Blessings Always Pauline (handwritten)

Pauline Gray, Ph.D., CNC

March 27, 2008 (handwritten)

Trafford
PUBLISHING

Order this book online at www.trafford.com/07-0525
or email orders@trafford.com

Most Trafford titles are also available at major online book retailers.

It is not the intent of the author to directly or indirectly diagnose, prescribe, provide medical advice
or replace a physician's care.

This book was written with the intent to educate the reader and to offer health information. In
the event you use this information without your doctors approval, you are prescribing for yourself,
which is your constitutional right.

Note for Librarians: A cataloguing record for this book is available from Library
and Archives Canada at www.collectionscanada.ca/amicus/index-e.html

Printed in Victoria, BC, Canada.

ISBN: 978-1-4251-2121-1

*We at Trafford believe that it is the responsibility of us all, as both individuals
and corporations, to make choices that are environmentally and socially sound.
You, in turn, are supporting this responsible conduct each time you purchase a
Trafford book, or make use of our publishing services. To find out how you are
helping, please visit www.trafford.com/responsiblepublishing.html*

*Our mission is to efficiently provide the world's finest, most comprehensive
book publishing service, enabling every author to experience success.
To find out how to publish your book, your way, and have it available
worldwide, visit us online at www.trafford.com/10510*

Trafford
PUBLISHING™ www.trafford.com

North America & international
toll-free: 1 888 232 4444 (USA & Canada)
phone: 250 383 6864 ♦ fax: 250 383 6804 ♦ email: info@trafford.com

The United Kingdom & Europe
phone: +44 (0)1865 722 113 ♦ local rate: 0845 230 9601
facsimile: +44 (0)1865 722 868 ♦ email: info.uk@trafford.com

10 9 8 7 6 5 4 3

TABLE OF CONTENTS

FORWARD

THE FOLLOWING IS THE synopsis of a man who has been in a ministry to assist the addicted for over 48 years. This author is honored and most appreciative of the time and consideration he has given to writing the forward for this book.

Most Sincerely,
Pauline Gray

In a world plagued by various addictions, I have tried many different theories and ideas to help people attain sobriety. In 1972, I became the chaplain at Albany County Jail and Mount McGregor Correctional Facility. I would hold these jobs for thirty years. During that time I established the Alcohol and Substance Abuse Program which would later on become the model for treatment in New York State Prisons. This program has grown from 20 clients to 41,000. I began to wonder how they would maintain sobriety, find work and housing once released from prison. Housing programs, which would also provide education, were developed throughout New York State.

To gain further insight, I went to Akron, Ohio and worked with Bill Wilson, the co-founder of Alcoholics Anonymous. This model (A.A.) was brought back with me to Albany, N.Y.

My ministry continues to grow. There are more that two dozen rehabilitation centers, halfway houses and alcohol crisis centers throughout New York State. I have ministered to alcoholics for 48 years and still open to ways to make each life better.

When Pauline Gray asked if I would consider writing the forward for her book, I was pleased to do so as I admire her work. Pauline Gray has provided some solid reasoning why we need to look at the "Wholistic Approach." This book covers and includes many major concerns for the professional counselor. The creative thinking she brings to the field about how it relates to teenagers, women, fetal alcohol syndrome and nutritional updates are essential for quality of treatment.

Reading the statistics about addiction and the numbers in this country that are devastated by this progressive and insidious disease is alarming, and yet it keeps growing. We need to be better informed, and Pauline Gray has done this in an easy to understand presentation.

We are currently meeting clients with co-occurring disorders. This book helps to clarify the relationship with Schizophrenia and alcohol. It explains that Schizophrenia is more than just a psychological disease. Also, new to many, will be the relationship between Hypoglycemia and medications that effect the success of our clients who are sick and suffering with their disease of addiction.

The final section of the book gets into a very practical approach toward diet. There are valuable guidelines and recommendations for delicious menus and suggestions for a nutrient balanced diet.

Working in this field, we are all aware of the damage that happens with the loss of essential nutrients during the drinking process.

I am impressed with Pauline Grays' work and recommend this book as an essential for all our clients.

Sincerely,

Father Peter G. Young

PREFACE

A NUTRITIONAL APPROACH TO THE TREATMENT OF ALCOHOLISM

THIS BOOK EXAMINES THE disease of alcoholism. As a professional who has worked with this populace since 1972, the author discusses how this problem has grown to monumental proportions. The book highlights biochemical rebalancing through proper nutrition versus pharmacology and hospital diets. It shows the development and delivery of services rendered to alcoholics and focuses on nutritional education for the treatment of alcoholism.

The disease of alcoholism presents a multitude of problems to the afflicted individual, family members, friends, neighbors, social service agencies and the public in general. Every life an alcoholic touches is affected by this disease in one fashion or another. The author has examined the problem of responding to the disease and the disturbance it creates for all who encounter it. This response suggests the importance of establishing facilities that meet the needs of the total person: mental, physical, spiritual and emotional. This book also responds to the need for family support and education regarding these areas.

The author has examined the obstacles presented by the community, families of alcoholics and to a no lesser degree, from the afflicted person involved. The authors' approach to documenting data critical to the developmental program is examined within the pages of this book. All reports and documents that have been compiled are based on the author's clinical experience with alcoholics, reports cited by the medical profession, interviews with former inmates of New York State Correctional Facilities, and long-time members of Alcoholics Anonymous. The documentation for this book also comes from the author's self-developed questionnaire, experiments with diet and supplementation of nutrients.

After compiling all of this information, the author felt justified to use the techniques described within these pages because all other programs had approached the alcoholic as either having a physical and/or mental problem and never took into consideration that they are the sum total of all their parts.

I

INTRODUCTION

THE DISEASE OF ALCOHOLISM has gained considerable notoriety in the United States. In terms of cause or treatment, whether it be psychological or physical, we still know little about this illness regardless of all the attention it receives. The intent of this book is to present research regarding pharmacology, and nutritional treatments, to address the specific concerns of those with the disease, to enhance the readers' understanding of the problems involved with the disease and finally, to show all readers that through counseling and biochemical rebalancing, there is life without alcohol.

Nutritional deficiencies and/or chemical imbalance may predispose individuals to this disease. Possible preventive measures may be taken from a nutritional point of view. As a nutritional consultant, it has been the author's experience that nutritional aid (both food and food supplements) has proven beneficial in the recovery process.

The author draws upon her personal experience working with alcoholics and demonstrates the importance of treating the alcoholic according to the nutritional needs of each individual in conjunction with psychological treatment.

Persons with the disease of alcoholism have very definite body, mind needs which require a program with a specialized staff and the education and cooperation of the surrounding community. Most programs of this kind have been met with adverse reaction in many communities. Adversity comes, for the most part, from lack of education and fear.

It is the author's belief that people with the disease of alcoholism require sufficient nutritional intervention and that the medical and psychological establishment has played the former down.

In her holistic scheme of thinking, the root of all health lies in maintaining the integrity of the body systems. Taking better care of the cellular environment, through proper nutrition, helps the body withstand stress. That fact, juxtaposed with the critical percentage who benefit from the wonders of modern medicine, make argument for a cooperative alliance doubly compelling.

This book hopes to validate the nutritional aspect of treatment of alcoholism. The subtle bodies (mental, physical and emotional) live under one roof and should be treated thusly.

ALCOHOLISM: DEFINITION

Dorland's Medical Dictionary defines alcoholism as follows: A chronic behavioral disorder manifested by repeated drinking of alcoholic beverages in excess of the dietary and social uses of the community and to an extent that interferes with the drinker's health or his social or economic functioning.

Simply put, alcoholism is a chronic illness marked by un-controlled consumption of alcoholic beverages. It compromises physical and psychological well-being and interferes with family and occupational responsibilities.

OVERVIEW

Alcoholism is a drinking disorder that becomes addictive. The disease is progressive and its' dependence can occur in a short period of time (five years) or take upwards to twenty-five years.

Stage 1—"Partying" without adverse effects

Stage 2—"Partying" with some adverse effects (staggering, hangover)

Stage 3—Greater quantities of alcohol required to get "the buzz," but now memory lapse follows the drinking episodes

Stage 4—Lack of control, binge drinking

When the alcohol intake is interrupted physical dependence reveals itself since alcohol affects all body systems.

Adrenal Glands—Due to stress on the body, breathing is ac-celerated and the rate of digestion is decreased.

Heart—Palpitation, labored breathing, myocardial infarc-tion and stroke can occur.

Liver—Prolonged drinking of alcohol can cause liver in-flammation, nausea, abdominal pain and hepatitis.

Pancreas—This gland is greatly affected by stress. Digestion of food becomes difficult and ineffective.

Since alcohol affects the central nervous system, consisting of the spinal cord and brain, adverse psychological symptoms are experienced during withdrawal. Anxiety, tension and hal-lucinations may develop.

There is no one definite cause of alcoholism; however, biochemical abnormalities may be present. Psychological factors may include the need to relieve stress and to lessen the anxiety of unresolved conflict within relationships. Stress is a large part of most everyone's life; therefore, social elements may include peer pressure, the availability of alcohol, and the attempt to become socially acceptable.

ALCOHOLISM: FACTS AND FICTION

It wasn't until 1940 that a minority of medical professionals came to the decision that alcoholism was a disease. However, they could not determine where this disease originated. Some physicians believed it began in the body. Others insisted it was a mental illness brought on by inherent weakness, lack of character or family instability. If the disease were truly mental, a psychologist would have tremendous success with patients. If it were strictly physiological, with all the prescription drugs available, alcoholism would have become a disease of the past. It has been viewed as a moral issue and a loss of spirituality. Alcoholism is all of these things.

To this very day, alcoholism is surrounded by misinformation, denial and uninformed opinion.

Fiction—A person cannot be an alcoholic if he/she is employed, has their own business, owns a home, raises a family or has social standing in the community.

Fact—Many affluent people are alcoholic. However, they can go on to lose their family and possessions if the drinking continues and the disease progresses.

Fiction—If a person drinks periodically, they are not nor will they become alcoholic.

Fact—It isn't what you drink, where you drink or why you are drinking. It's all about what happens to you when you drink.

Fiction—Drinking wine will thin the blood.

Fact—Alcohol, in any form clogs the veins and arteries. This, in turn, increases the blood pressure.

Fiction—Drinking wine, brandy or beer will not cause a person to become an alcoholic.

Fact—It's all the same. By any other name, alcohol is alcohol. The chemical effect is no different.

Fiction—Only low income, uneducated, criminal types become alcoholics.

Fact—Margaret's case (chapter 3) shows otherwise. Financial status, education and moral character are all irrelevant. You cannot talk or buy your way out of the disease.

Fiction—In the right place, at the right time, an alcoholic can be shamed into abstinence.

Fact—No amount of ridicule or embarrassment will stop an alcoholic from drinking. If anything, it will provoke an all-out binge.

Fiction—All alcoholics "hit bottom."

Fact—Some are fortunate enough to recognize their problem and receive early intervention.

Fiction—Being dry means you're sober.

Fact—Mental clarity, emotional stability, a sense of peace and well-being, this adds up to sobriety.

The following story gives credence to this fact.

COOKIE AGE 28

When I looked in the mirror, I saw what I wanted to see. I was young, well rounded, smart. I was going to do something with my life, not waste it like my mother did. There were eleven of us kids in the family. My mother knocked herself out for us.

My father was home just long enough to make another kid and he was gone. We hardly ever saw him. He worked, drank, and came home to sleep it off.

My mother looked ten years older than she really was. That wasn't in the cards for me. I wasn't going to sit around with a house full of kids, washing dirty clothes and dishes all day.

When I turned seventeen, I left and got married. I got myself a job and at nineteen I started drinking. My drinking helped me with my confidence on the job. When I couldn't cope at work, I drank. Some mornings I'd crawl out of bed and be in the bathroom with diarrhea or vomiting. Sometimes both. I went to work anyway. The job was providing the money for my booze.

Soon there was no more job and no access to money for my alcohol. So what, I'd get another job. When the arguments started at home and things got out of hand, my husband walked out. So what, there were plenty more where he came from. My mother soon became "the enabler." I'd go over to her house and carry on about how nobody understood how tough things were for me. She'd give me the money, either out of fear or, to get this argumentative alcoholic out of her house.

I drank when I was happy, sad, alone or in a crowd. I wound up, flat on my back, at a rehabilitation center. SO WHAT. In and out of rehabs, job after job, man after man. I still didn't get the picture because I was doing what I wanted. I wasn't stuck at home with a bunch of kids like my mother. I really thought my life was better than hers.

What a joke. Nothing was better, it was just different.

When I wasn't drinking, I considered myself sober. Yet, I was depressed, had an explosive temper and mood swings. This went on for years. Finally, I admitted my alcohol addiction. It had great power over me. I thank the members of Alcoholics Anonymous, my doctor and nutritional consultant for their intervention, support and continued encouragement. I couldn't have done it on my own. I found out, the hard way, that being dry doesn't necessarily mean being sober.

VARIOUS MODALITIES

Alcoholism is complex and challenges health care providers to alleviate both the symptoms and consequences of alcohol abuse and dependence. They need to consider the clinical pharmacology of alcohol, the pathogenesis (the cellular events and reactions occurring in the development of the disease), diagnosis, management and complications of the addiction. All clinicians should continue learning how to care for the alcoholic patient especially the difficult cases. The management of withdrawal and recovery is dealt with inconsistency and at times in a contradictory way. Take the following clients case for example.

ED AGE 46

Ed had a long history of alcohol abuse. He drank over a period of twenty six years. During that time he was in and out of recovery, spent thirty days in jail (twice), and six months in jail (three times). Nothing changed for him. Over the years, various medications were administered. Each had a temporary effect. Ed eventually was sent to Hudson Correctional Facility, Hudson, New York. It was there he was introduced to Alcoholics Anonymous for the first time. He spent a total of twenty three months in Hudson. Ed did well under constant supervision, but was not taught how to adapt to the outside world regarding his addiction.

He was released and was out only eight months when he was admitted to the V.A. Hospital Rehabilitation Unit in Albany, New York. There he was given blood tests to determine any deficiencies and the proper food supplements to correct any imbalance. After thirty days, he returned home and stayed clean for sixteen months, only to do another six months at a half-way house. There was no medication administered, no blood work or supplements, and residents prepared their own meals. The only restriction placed on them was daily A.A. meetings and curfew. However, Ed is a success story. Shortly after his release, Ed became a client of the author. He was faithful attending A.A. meetings, mindful of the food he ate, and took appropriate food supplements to meet his individual need. Ed exercises five times a week and has taken up bowling for relaxation. He no longer falls prey to peer pressure and balances his life with work, play and rest. Ed is proud to say, "April 3, 2007, I am sober nine years."

Having read Ed's story, we see how treatments vary from facility to facility with no continuity or consistency. How then will each clinician continue to approach physical and psychological issues that contribute to and exacerbate alcoholism? Are we prepared for the toll this drinking disorder will take on future generations without furthering our knowledge?

The following pages contain various modalities currently being used for the treatment of alcoholism.

ACUPUNCTURE

Acupuncture originated in China more than five thousand years ago. It is based on the belief that health is determined by the flow of vital energy within all living organisms.

According to theory, this energy travels through twelve major pathways known as meridians. Each pathway corresponds to a specific organ or gland. Special needles are used and inserted just below the skin to help rebalance the flow of energy, thus restoring health.

Regarding its popularity, it is widely used in America as an effective treatment for alcohol addiction. Acupuncture views addiction as an imbalance in the flow of this vital energy.

Due to its success, many state judiciary systems offer it as part of their health care and encourage further development. The Wayne County jail in Detroit, Michigan has such a program.

CHIROPRACTIC

Chiropractics' concern is the relationship of the spinal column to the nervous system. It was formally introduced in 1895.

Sir Jay Holder, D.C., of Miami, Florida explains, "The nervous system holds the key to the body's incredible potential to heal itself because it coordinates and controls the functions of all the other systems of the body."

By adjusting the spine to remove subluxation, normal nerve function may be restored.

Dr. Holder has worked with the University of Miami School of Medicine conducting a study to prove the effectiveness of Chiropractic adjustment with addiction.

GUIDED IMAGERY

Guided imagery uses the power of the mind to evoke positive thoughts to create well-being. Through these thoughts a person can see, feel, smell, taste and/or hear in ones' imagination. Breathing exercises and other relaxation techniques are used to quiet the mind and body to maximize this imagery.

Imagery soothes the body, mind and emotion. It can facilitate recovery, enable people to cope more effectively and come to grips with their life.

Martin L. Rossman, M.D., co-founder of the Academy of Imagery refers to it as, "The language of the emotions and the interface between body and mind."

Taught properly, it is a great tool for increasing self-esteem and self-control.

YOGA

Yoga is an ancient art of self-improvement. It is one of the oldest systems of health and dates back five thousand years. Hatha Yoga (physical postures), Raja Yoga (breathing techniques) and meditation practice have proven successful in reducing stress. Since stress is such a large part of everyone's life today, practicing yoga for only this one reason would prove highly beneficial.

The practitioner learns to regulate autonomic function such as heart and respiration. Through the postures, breathing techniques and meditation, physical tension fades. Yoga helps a person get in touch with the body and feelings; to comprehend situations clearly and cope more effectively.

The mind/body benefits of yoga are far reaching. Hatha Yoga addresses all body systems: circulatory, digestive, glandular, immune, intestinal and nervous. Incorporating Raja Yoga with the Hatha practice furthers the benefits by including the respiratory and lymphatic systems.

The Yoga Biomedical Trust charted the response of alcoholics who were prescribed yoga as an alternative treatment therapy. One hundred percent claimed benefit.

Adopting one or more of the aforementioned modalities as part of a program would be an important addition to alcoholism treatment.

2

ALCOHOLISM AMONG TEENAGERS

THE DRINKING DISORDER OF alcoholism has reached epidemic proportions throughout the world. In the United States alone, the number of reported cases is staggering. Statistics show there are over 14 million alcoholics, of which, nearly 10 million are teenagers who drink alcohol weekly.

According to the National Council on Alcoholism, "Alcohol is America's No. 1 drug problem among youth." Adolescents, ages 9 through 19, are experiencing negative consequences of alcohol abuse—impairment of health or school performance, involvement in an accident, arrest and incarceration. Each year approximately 10,000 young people between the ages of 16 and 24 are killed in alcohol related accidents, including suicides, homicides and violent injuries. Alcohol related highway deaths are the No. 1 killer of 15 to 24 year olds.

Early drinking increases lifetime injury risks. Ralph

Hingson, Sc.D., reports in the Journal of the American Medical Association, "The younger people are when they begin drinking, the more likely they are to be injured under the influence of alcohol." Dr. Hingson's analysis for the injury risk study was supported by the National Highway Administration.

According to the Department of Justice, "Alcohol consumption is associated with 27 percent of all murders, 33 percent of all property offenses, and more than 37 percent of the young people in adult correctional facilities reported drinking before committing a crime."

Statistics further show children of alcoholics have a four times greater risk of developing alcoholism than children of non-alcoholics.

Parents and the public in general show concern about the use of drugs in schools, and rightly so, but alcohol is twice as popular among high school and college students and five times more popular than cocaine. Two reasons for this may be cost and availability.

As if alcohol addiction wasn't enough, a far more reaching problem prevails among our youth today. The area of involvement is not the disease of alcoholism alone, but a cross or dual addiction. The earlier in life a person begins using alcohol the more likely it is he or she will experiment and go on to use other drugs. This compounds the problem leading to multiple health and social problems.

Despite the fact that alcohol impairs judgement, alcohol is treated differently from other drugs. Alcohol is encouraged at social events and when an individual becomes intoxicated, they are generally viewed as comical. Alcoholic beverages are readily accessible and reasonably priced, making it the drug of choice.

Alcoholic is a word most people are uncomfortable with, but when you are young, it's that much more difficult. When one youth was confronted about the use of alcohol and its' potential danger he had this to say, "You gotta be kiddin me. I have some beers on the weekend, maybe a few shots. I'm no alcoholic, I'm havin some fun. Get over it."

Teenagers and pre-teens need to be taught alcoholism does not discriminate. It is an illness which effects young and old alike, rich, poor, black, white, yellow, red and any color in between. The fact beer is chosen over hard liquor doesn't matter and it doesn't make a difference in the length of time a person drinks. The bottom line is—what happens to a person when they drink.

Drinking can spin one's universe out of control. It creates problems in the home with parents, at school causing grades to spiral downward, missed days and job loss. One drink alters the body and mind, thus reducing stress and making a person feel more liked by their peers. But, alcohol is a drug, causing addiction. When the party is over and the sun rises, the same problems exist. Perhaps they are compounded due to the need for alcohol.

Drinking alcohol allows a person to take risks they might never take. It frees inhibitions and the quiet person soon becomes the life of the party. It now gives them the courage to ask that cute girl or cool guy for a dance. The usually friendly person may become loud and obnoxious. With intoxication comes reckless decision making—unprotected sex, trying illicit drugs and the drive home. Alcohol use has been the cause of date rape, battery and homicide.

What other fate does alcohol abuse have for the teenager? Let's begin by saying, "Alcohol poisons the body systems when too much is consumed too quickly." It causes vomiting, stomach ulcers (which may bleed), blackouts, cirrhosis of the liver and mental illness.

Most teenagers think this could never happen to them because with youth comes invincibility. The aforementioned only happens to "old folks."

Many teenagers develop into healthy adults despite the fact being a teenager has never been easy, but this chapter isn't about them. It's about those adolescents who constantly feel the stress to win their parents approval, to get good grades (or just pass), to be popular. Countless teenagers are living through their own special crisis—physical or verbal abuse in the home, divorce, never having had a father figure, alcoholic/drug addicted parent(s) or financial hardship.

Unfortunately, there are those times when personal pressures compounded by alcohol cause serious emotional problems for some teenagers. This is the time when the parent(s), teachers, and health care professionals need to intervene. Learning about and recognizing symptoms of mental illness at its' onset would make it more treatable and preventive.

Alcohol and drug abuse, anxiety, depression, obsessive-compulsive behavior and physical abuse are a few disorders of our youth today. Responsible adults need to be mindful of such problems.

Too many teenagers are drinking and for them, alcoholism is on the rise. It not only is affecting their lives today, it also affects their future. The following interviews give sound argument for early intervention.

CINDY AGE 16

Three years ago I was in Junior High. I was hanging out with some of my friends. One of the girls heard about this party and got us invited. It was a Friday and sounded like a great way to start the weekend.

When I got home, I asked my folks if it was okay. They wanted to know if the parents would be at home. I said yes even though I didn't really know. My folks said it was okay with them as long as I was home by 10:30. My girlfriends stopped by around 7:30 and off we went, not knowing what was in store.

When we got to the party, there was a bunch of people there. Looking around, I could see that a lot of them were high school seniors. This was a first for me, hanging out with the older guys. I admit, I was excited. It made me feel grownup. I wasn't in the house a long time, when I noticed there were no parents, and the older guys had brought alcohol. After awhile, the place started to have a peculiar odor. One of my friends mentioned guys and girls were in the other room smoking "weed." I promised myself I'd stay clear of that area.

I was standing around when one of the older guys asked me if I wanted a beer. "I don't like beer, thanks." He walked away, but came back a little while later with a mixed drink. It tasted really good. I can't say, to this day, how many more of those drinks I had. I do know I wound up in the other room smoking "weed." I vaguely remember winding up in bed with some bozo. His face is still a blur. Then along came a guy who I thought was my savior.

Luke, a senior, got me out of there. He helped me to his car cause I couldn't make it on my own. My friends??? Who cared. I was out of it. I realize now, we were about ten minutes from my house when Luke passed out behind the wheel of his car. When I woke up I saw bright lights, cops, and a man holding a hysterical woman. "Where the heck am I?" "You're in the emergency room," some voice said. I didn't even know what happened. I later found out that Luke went off the road into a tree. He died instantly. As for me, I've been sitting in this wheel chair for three years and will continue to sit here for the rest of my life.

My life, as it could have been, is over. Do I have a message? You bet I do. My message to everyone who reads this story is this: It was my first party without my parents. It was the very first time I drank alcohol and my first time trying a drug. I learned too late to think before doing something stupid.

Did Cindy's parents ever sit with her to explain the hazards of drinking alcohol and taking drugs? Were the dangers of alcohol abuse taught in her school? Do we know if this tragedy could have been prevented?

Many questions go unanswered. Although Cindy has been in therapy for two years, she refuses to discuss life at home. She does say, "My parents are divorced because my father couldn't handle it." This leaves room for speculation regarding the family dynamics.

ARNIE AGE 19

Arnie was separated from his family and was sleeping in his friends basement. How did that come about? He stopped going to school, laid around the house all day and gave his mother grief. His father got sick of it, opened the door and as Arnie says, "My old man kicked me in the butt and told me to get a job." Arnie wasn't going to flip burgers and make French fries all day. He got together with some friends in the neighborhood to make some fast money.

It was Halloween night. The three sat around Joey's basement drinking beer, then rum and coke. They were all pretty drunk when Joey started talking about the liquor store on Green

Street and how the old guy was always alone when he closed up. They thought it would be an easy way to pick up more liquor and quick cash. Arnie was concerned about getting caught.

They took Joey's father's car and drove down. Joey had put baseball bats in the back seat of the car. He said it was a bad neighborhood and they might have to protect themselves. It was supposed to be a fast in and out. They would grab some bottles, get the cash and be home free. Then, party time back at Joey's house. They went in, bats in hand.

The owner of the store thought they were there to buy liquor and wouldn't sell it to them because they were under age. Joey got angry. Arnie and Frankie began to panic. They grabbed the bottles and cash. There was a struggle and Mr. A. (the store owner) was beat without mercy. As they fled from the store and rounded the corner, a patrol car was approaching. They jumped into their car and sped off with the patrol car in pursuit. The chase went on for twenty minutes. The three adolescents were arrested and brought to justice. Arnie blamed the whole incident on the alcohol.

Mrs. A usually met her husband at closing time, but decided to stay home that night for the trick or treaters. It's a night, she says, she'll never forget. When the doorbell rang, she picked up the bowl of candy, opened the door and was met by a policeman with the news of her husband's tragic death.

This story is close to the author's heart. It was told to her by Mrs. A., a dear friend.

BRIAN AGE 17

Brian's mother had him in and out of therapy since he was twelve years old. He always seemed depressed, didn't do well with relationships and dropped out of school. He'd roll out of bed at noon, grab a pepsi, then watch T.V. for hours. He had no plans for his future. His mother and live-in boyfriend never saw Brian drink alcohol or use drugs. However, by the time they got home from work, Brian was already gone and didn't get in until one or two in the morning.

It was a Saturday in May of 2003. Brian took the loaded gun his "stepfather" kept in the dresser drawer. He robbed the local convenience store two miles from his house. His motive— money for alcohol and cocaine.

Brian entered the store. There was no one there except the young clerk behind the counter. Seeing Brian's gun, the clerk was more than willing to empty the cash drawer. Brian left, picked up his alcohol and drugs as planned.

Brian's mother got home from work after finishing her shift at the hospital. Not expecting Brian to be home, she didn't call out to him. After a few minutes, she noticed a scratching noise coming from Brian's bedroom. Thinking he had accidentally locked the cat in the room, she opened the door. Her son lie on the floor in a pool of blood. Alcohol bottles were strewn about. There was a gun nearby and the side of his face was completely blown off.

Looking back, Brian's mother remembers how peaceful he appeared in spite of the tragedy.

She went on to reveal her own alcohol dependence in the past.

Adolescents are being lost to alcohol and drug abuse. The correctional facilities are filled to capacity with tragic stories.

The information in this chapter and those that follow is important. Hopefully it will heighten the awareness of the afflicted, parents, teachers, physicians and other health care providers.

3

ALCOHOL AND WOMEN

YEARS AGO, MEN WERE known to drink alcohol more than women. Therefore, it was the female counterpart who was more likely to experience alcoholism. However, in the past twenty years, drinking differences between men and women has diminished. In relation to the amount consumed and the problems encountered, the gap has narrowed considerably.

In June 2000, a government survey suggested, "Fifty three percent of women who are more than occasional drinkers are problem drinkers i.e. they experience problems of psychological and/or physical dependence."

CAROL LYNN AGE 55
"I've always taken pride in my personal appearance, always wanting to present a nice image. When I first started drinking

and had a late night, I could always manage to bounce back and look perky the next day. As my drinking got worse, I'd wake in the morning looking a little older, a little more tired, and a lot more bloated. I'd have a beer for breakfast, put on my makeup (a little extra) and feel fine. Gradually, that wasn't working for me anymore. It got to be more booze, a whole lot more makeup and soon, who the hell cared. Not me."

As progression began, Carol Lynn displayed signs of tension, nervousness and outbursts of temper. In the advanced stage of drinking alcohol, her body/mind gave way to weakness and depressive mental states.

People have been known to think of the alcoholic as a person having had many disadvantages in their life. Thereby exposed to a life of poverty and hopelessness. The fact is, Carol Lynn exceeded average grades in school and was known as a perfectionist. She was successful in her endeavors and carried out chores at all cost. This personality trait carried over into her personal life. The enthusiastic response she had toward work, etc. she now expected from friends and family members. When others did not meet with her expectations, she became verbally abusive. To cope with what she saw as a lack of cooperation a few drinks were taken at lunchtime. Later, she began to drink to "unwind" at the end of a hectic day. The drinking escalated. The disease progressed. Her alcohol consumption increased regardless of cost. Carol Lynn stated many times, "I can quit any time." But, it took over her life. At one point, she became so overwhelmed by the disease, she prayed for death. For too many, this happens.

The heaviest female drinkers of alcohol appear to be those between the ages of 16-24. Women who drink heavily usually engage in a very active social life which involves alcohol consumption. With the women's liberation movement came changes in the attitude, status and position of women in society. This made drinking alcohol for women socially acceptable.

In recent years, the media has portrayed alcohol consumption as sexual, glamorous, a desirable lifestyle. If drinking alcohol is more socially acceptable than the use of marijuana and/or cocaine, "Is alcoholism a social disease?" In the book Psycho-Dietetics, Mercedes McCambridge (former actress and recovered alcoholic) says, "Alcoholics aren't evil or immoral. I've been one. Alcoholism is a disease that effects body, mind, spirit and that is the disaster.

Most women are at greater risk for alcohol related problems than men. In a large portion of violent crimes, women are particularly vulnerable due to another persons alcohol abuse. In more than half of the violent crimes perpetrated on women, sexual assault and rape, the assailant was found to be intoxicated. Studies have shown, at the time of the offense, the victims were also under the influence of alcohol.

Women suffer physical and psychosocial harm at lower levels of drinking than men. This may be due to the fact women have lower levels of ADH (Alcohol Dehydrogenase). ADH is an enzyme required for alcohol metabolism.

PROBLEMS SPECIAL TO WOMEN

The increase of alcohol consumption puts women at risk for special problems.

Breast Cancer—Alcohol is associated with a higher risk of breast cancer. Drinking excessive amounts may be a predisposing factor. The Nurses Health Survey reported that women drinking more than three glasses of wine per day increased the risk of developing breast cancer by up to three times.

Liver Disease—Women develop liver disease (hepatitis and Cirrhosis) in a shorter period of time than men. This may be due, in part, to the fact that women have a higher ration of fat versus water in the system. This makes the female less able to dilute the alcohol thus, allowing for higher concentration of alcohol in the blood.

PREGNANCY AND SUBSTANCE ABUSE

Alcohol consumption during pregnancy has the potential of damaging two people. It is a major problem confronting obstetrics today. The deleterious effects on the unborn child raise many medical questions.

Physicians, nutritionists and counselors need to educate the pregnant woman who requires help confronting her problem. Women who abuse alcohol often abuse other substances such as tobacco and/or illegal drugs. The impact of dual addiction must be taken into account when evaluating the effects of these substances on the unborn child. Obstetrics complications may be intensified by malnutrition, alcohol and cigarette abuse and sexually transmitted diseases.

Alcohol and cigarettes are the substances most widely used during pregnancy. A National Pregnancy and Health Survey revealed: "At least 800,000 women smoke cigarettes and 757,000 drink alcohol during their pregnancy." Many of these women continue to drink alcohol to avoid withdrawal symptoms. However, many women continue drinking alcohol not knowing the danger involved.

Since alcohol and drug addiction carry a social stigma, the

female patient tends to minimize their substance abuse, giving inaccurate information. Physicians need to establish a trusting relationship with their patient. This opens the lines of communication to reveal dependence. Proper care and intervention can not take place without admission of the abuse.

FETAL ALCOHOL SYNDROME

DEFINITION

Syndrome—A set of symptoms which occur together; the sum of signs of any morbid state.

Fetal Alcohol Syndrome—A symptom of altered prenatal growth occurring in infants born of women who were chronically alcoholic during pregnancy.

These symptoms include

1 Prominence of the forehead and lower jaw

2 Palpebral (eyelid) fissures

3 Microphthalmia (abnormal smallness in one or both eyes)

4 Severe growth and mental retardation

5 Microcephaly (abnormal smallness of the head)

6 Central nervous dysfunction

Fetal abnormalities were described as early as 1968, but it was not referred to as "fetal alcohol syndrome" until 1973 when the pattern of malformation was cited in the Lancet.

There is no specific data which shows at which level of drinking this harm occurs. Therefore, physicians should encourage patients to abstain from drinking alcohol since there is possibly no safe level.

Education is the first step in intervention. A one-on-one discussion with a trusted physician and nutritional consultant can be very effective for recovery from alcoholism. Patients who require additional treatment should be given the appropriate referrals.

Society has been led to believe female alcoholism occurs only in low income areas, amongst uneducated people. As stated previously, alcoholism does not discriminate. A perfect example of this follows.

MARGARET AGE 35

Margaret was popular in school. She was well liked, president of her class, a cheer leader and wrote for the school newspaper.

She graduated high school with honors, continued on to college, carried a 3.9 grade average and graduated Medical School. Several years later, she went into private practice with a former classmate. The two were unsinkable. They put in long hours and were greatly admired by their patients.

There were nights when Margaret could not "come down" from the events of the day. She began taking an occasional night cap. She'd wake the next morning all ready to go. Barbara, her colleague, never suspected what was going on. Margaret kept her secret well hidden.

Margaret became romantically involved, but never revealed her alcohol problem to her new husband. Her alcohol abuse managed to go undetected for quite some time until the illness progressed and various problems began to surface. With the love and support of her husband Jim, Margaret attended Alcoholics Anonymous. On the nights he didn't go to the meeting with her, Margaret would leave the meeting and head straight for a local club. She'd arrive home late and pass out on the bed.

There were many appointments missed and Barbara was beginning to take on the extra load at the office. Margaret promised Barbara it wouldn't happen again. In order to function, Margaret added amphetamines to her alcohol. She wrote her own prescriptions under patients names. Everything came to a head. Margaret left her medical practice.

After several months at home Margaret became pregnant, but never stopped drinking. Her behavior was outrageous. Jim insisted she go to a rehabilitation center to detoxify.

Margaret gave birth to a baby girl. Claire weighed 3 pounds 6 ounces. After Margaret was released from the hospital she went on a binge, the likes of which Jim had never seen.

When Claire weighed enough to come home, Jim packed his things, took the baby and moved out. There were legal battles and financial ruin. Jim got total custody of Claire. Margaret's practice was gone, her marriage destroyed, she lost her child and life as she formerly knew it vanished.

THE WORD ON CLAIRE

Alcohol and amphetamines damaged Claire while in the womb. She was diagnosed with FAS and required special attention. She has tremors, a short attention span and is tiny for her age. The energy it takes to care for this child is exhausting.

If Margaret had abused her child after birth the way she did during her pregnancy, she would have gone before a Judge, charged with reckless endangerment and spend time incarcerated in a correctional facility.

No one can say Margaret drank from ignorance or that she was socially or economically deprived.

4

SCHIZOPHRENIA AND ALCOHOL

SCHIZOPHRENIA IS A SEVERE emotional disorder characterized by delusions, hallucinations, regressive or bizarre behavior. Some patients may appear normal, but suddenly lash out for no apparent reason. Schizophrenia has erroneously been called "split personality."

The number of Schizophrenic alcoholics are growing in leaps and bounds. The New York State Commission for the Mentally Disabled says, "There are more than 100,000 such dually disabled psychiatric patients in New York State alone. The mentally ill are the most visible of the alcoholics. They are the most likely to be homeless, and most likely to end up in jail after committing a drug related crime."

The father of a Schizophrenic alcoholic states, "The alcoholism programs can deal with the alcoholic. The mental health programs can deal with mental illness. My son has both and they haven't got a clue how to deal with him."

Ironically, they eat up a large share of the systems resources even though effective programs for treating them have yet to be developed. This population makes up a significant portion of admissions to the psychiatric facilities in many states. Once they are stabilized, they are discharged because there is no further program for them. They fail in the community and end up being readmitted to the psychiatric ward or left to wander the city streets.

Although hospitals in New York State have set up programs to treat mentally ill alcoholics, one of the fundamental difficulties in developing such a program is, "Mental health professionals and substance abuse counselors use diametrically opposed treatment."

Over the past ten years, the State of New York has spent millions of dollars to develop a program. In 1992, Kathleen Sciacca, director of Substance Abuse Programs, Wingdale, New York found some sort of solution for the mentally ill alcoholic. On her own initiative, she developed a treatment approach which emphasized educating patients on the effects of alcohol and drug abuse, using therapy groups that encourage patients to support each other emotionally. She didn't have them immediately admit their addictions, stop drinking or using drugs. She noted, "Many clients have made progress. So far these patients have remained out of the hospital for longer periods of time and were able to attend a series of Alcoholics Anonymous meetings. They formerly were disruptive at A.A. meetings. They also remained abstinent from substance abuse."

Hospitals, clinics and programs have become involved. However, the influence Biochemical Rebalancing, by way of nutrition, may have on this disease receives little consideration.

A person who neglects his/her essential dietary needs can be nothing other than malnourished. This in itself causes metabolic disturbances which manifest in countless ways. Many schizophrenics experience nutritional disease. Some curtail their eating habit so severely they have been treated for pellagra.

Evidence has been presented of an abnormal biochemical profile in individuals with psychological disorders. Many of these parameters are related to dietary intake. Cause and effect relationships exist. Hormonal imbalance can lead to gross behavioral distortion. A fact well established is the influence of diet upon the endocrine glands. The schizophrenic's behavior may be due, in part, to a metabolic disorder related to nutritional deficiencies. The same applies to the alcoholic.

Over the past several decades, biochemistry has given considerable insight in understanding human behavior. Schizophrenia by itself is destructive; think of the complexity surrounding the Schizophrenic alcoholic. These people are stumbling through life. Many of them are not ill enough to be hospitalized, and not well enough to live in the community.

Schizophrenia has three primary etiologic factors: heredity, stress and constitutional defense mechanism. However, every case cannot be explained on any one hypothesis, and a single cause of schizophrenia has not been found. There is evidence that the schizophrenias include a group characterized by an impairment of the homeostatic control mechanisms situated in the hypothalamus.

THE SYMPTOMS OF SCHIZOPHRENIA

Schizophrenics experience depression, hear voices and see things in a distorted fashion. The sense of smell, taste, sound and sight are lost. Compound this with the side effects of alcoholism and you have a person who appears demented.

The following defines the perceptual changes and personality alterations most frequently experienced:

Visual—Illusions and hallucinations, people and objects appear distorted. The real blends with the unreal.

Auditory—Buzzing, hissing, a whisper may be deafening, a shout not heard.

Sense of Smell—Strong odors fade: sweet odors may be malodorous.

Sense of Touch—Crawling sensations: a gentle touch may be painful, a body slam not felt.

Taste—Poisons are suspected in foods: Familiar food tastes strange.

Mood—Deep, almost continual depression, irrational fear and extreme tension

Behavior—Outbursts of violence for no apparent reason: suicide attempts, eccentric emotional attachments

The following is an account of a client who has made great progress.

DOROTHY AGE 57

"I'm an alcoholic, diagnosed with schizophrenia. For more years than I care to remember, I was addicted to valium and Librium. I also found myself popping amphetamines to counteract the drowsiness from the other drugs. When I drank, I got very aggressive and was arrested seven times for assault. I was in the hospital many times and at one point got shock therapy. Things got real bad for me so I went to a rehab. I thought I was doing pretty good, but after I got out I found myself having hallucinations even without touching a drink. I was so damned depressed with my life, I hit the bottle. God knows I couldn't hold down a job and my family gave up on me a long time ago. Now, I'm okay."

Dorothy tried attending A.A. meetings, but was too disruptive. A friend of hers had contacted the author asking if she could help. Nutritional counseling was suggested along with a whole foods diet similar to the one appearing later in this book. Dorothy was found to have hypoglycemia and was asked to remove all sugar and white flour products from her diet. Within several months of eating well and taking the suggested nutritional food supplements, Dorothy was well enough to attend regular A.A. meetings without a problem. Her drinking has stopped for the first time in many years and she celebrates her sobriety.

MORE THAN A PSYCHOLOGICAL DISEASE

Alcohol is a powerful drug. It affects the adrenal glands, brain, central nervous system, gall bladder, gastrointestinal tract, liver, pancreas and skin. Alcohol can be seen as a narcotic that impairs the overall health of any individual. The following pages address various organs, glands and body parts and their relationship to alcohol consumption.

THE ADRENAL GLANDS

The body has two adrenal glands. Each adrenal gland is positioned superior to each kidney. These have been called the "fight or flight" glands. Stress, due to consistent intake of alcohol, greatly affects the adrenal glands. Under stress conditions, impulses are received by the brain to increase the output of epinephrine and norepinephrine. Epinephrine increases blood pressure by increasing the heart rate and force of constriction and by constricting the blood vessels. It accelerates the rate of respiration, dilates the respiratory passageways, decreases the rate of digestion, increases the efficiency of muscular contractions, increases blood sugar levels and stimulates cellular metabolism.

ALCOHOL AND THE BRAIN

When alcohol reaches the brain, the first part to become affected is the frontal lobe. This is the reasoning part of the brain. As the alcohol continues to enter the bloodstream, the speech and vision center of the brain become involved. The third area are the cells of the brain that control the large muscles. At this point, a person begins to stagger. Alcohol not only interferes with normal brain function, but destroys the cells in the process.

The blood carries oxygen and nutrients to the brain. Since the brain uses 25% of carbohydrates for fuel, a diet low in complex carbohydrates causes glucose starvation. Alcohol disrupts oxygen and glucose metabolism causing dizziness, mental confusion and even unconsciousness.

There are two essential B vitamins required to convert glucose to energy, B1 and B3. Alcohol soaks up the B vitamins like a sponge soaks up water, leaving the brain cells lacking in glucose energy.

Polyneuropathy, a disease which involves several nerves, and Korsakoff's psychosis are severe complications resulting from these vitamin deficiencies. Korsakoff is accompanied by disturbance of orientation, susceptibility to external stimulation and suggestion, amnesia, hallucinations and especially confabulation (imaginary experiences). Wernicke's Syndrome is caused by a thiamine (B1) deficiency, with alcoholism as a contributing factor. Mental changes range from forgetfulness to delirium tremens (DT's).

PAULINE GRAY

HEART

Alcoholic Cardiomyopathy is caused by excessive use of alcohol. Alcohol abuse acts directly upon the cell membranes in the heart muscle, having a toxic effect. The result is poor heart function. Alcoholic Cardiomyopathy is usually seen in males 35 to 55 years of age, but has been known to effect older patients.

One of the major causes of death in alcoholics is heart failure. Two of the symptoms are heart palpitation and labored breathing. Death results from cardiac arrhythmia, myocardial infarction and stroke.

Interviews with 2,170 men under the age of 55 experiencing their first non-fatal myocardial infarction revealed: "Those who drank 1 to 7 times per week had a relative risk of 1.2 compared to non-drinkers. These studies did not support previous studies which claimed that moderate consumption of alcohol reduced the risk of developing myocardial infarction."

THE LIVER

The liver is a major organ which, among other functions, converts fat into energy. When alcohol is in the body, it can either convert the alcohol or the fat for energy. Since alcohol is the easier of the two for conversion, the liver quickly makes its' selection. The fat is then kept in storage.

"Liver cells prefer fatty acids as their fuel. When alcohol is present, the cells are forced to use alcohol. The fatty acids then accumulate in huge stockpiles."

If conditions in the liver last long enough, cells die and the area will be invaded by scar tissue. The end result is called fibrosis. Biochemical rebalancing, through good nutrition, and abstinence from alcohol can reverse the fibrosis.

If the liver becomes swollen and inflamed, hepatitis is experienced. The alcoholic runs high fevers, feels nauseated, has abdominal pain and jaundice. This too can be reversed.

If, after all of this, the individual continues to abuse their body with alcohol, they may encounter an irreversible liver disease known as cirrhosis. The scar tissue in the liver now constricts the blood vessels. When the blood can no longer circulate freely through the fatty, congested, scarred liver, the pressure created will now cause the small blood vessels in the face to rupture. This results in spider-like patterns called Spider Angioma.

ALCOHOLS AFFECT ON THE PANCREAS

The pancreas is a large gland, six to eight inches long, lying crosswise in the upper posterior portion of the abdomen. It secretes enzymes (chemicals) into the intestines for the digestion of foods. Chronic alcoholism creates a severe stress situation in the body. The pancreas is greatly affected by stress. As the disease of alcoholism progresses, the digestion of foods is ineffective. Eventually, a lack of enzyme conversion results from the body's constant onslaught of alcohol. This leads to heartburn, gastritis and bloating. Pancreatitis (inflammation of the pancreas) can develop. This is associated with indigestion and foul smelling stools.

A major function of the pancreas is blood sugar regulation. An internal secretion, insulin, is produced in the beta cells. Insulin is concerned with the regulation of carbohydrate metabolism and decreased blood sugar levels.

Glucagon, a polypeptide hormone, is produced in the alpha cells. Both the alpha and the beta cells form aggregates called "islets of Langerhans." Glucagon's principle activity is to increase the blood sugar level. This action is performed by converting glycogen into glucose in the liver. The liver releases the glucose into the bloodstream and the blood sugar level rises. It is important to note the interaction between the liver and the pancreas.

THE ARTERIES

Another of the many common conditions afflicting the untreated alcoholic is hypertension (high blood pressure). This is defined as consistently high arterial pressure. Three particular types are associated with alcoholism.

Portal hypertension—Frequent complication of cirrhosis of the liver.

Secondary hypertension—Associated with disorders of the central nervous system and endocrine diseases.

Splenoportal—Results from an obstruction of the splenic venous system resulting from enlargement of the liver.

Hypertension is considered a major risk factor for stroke.

As far back as 1953, the Honolulu Heart Program studied 8,006 men living on the island of Oahu. This report is based on a twelve year follow-up. During that period of time, there were 93 strokes among non-drinkers and 197 strokes among drinkers. The incidence of stroke was almost five times higher for heavy drinkers as non-drinkers. After adjustment for other risk factors, such as smoking and high blood pressure, drinkers still had 2 to 3 times as much risk as non-drinkers, and the risk was greater for heavy and moderate drinkers than for light drinkers.

When people reduce their alcohol consumption, they lower their risk of developing stroke significantly.

URINARY SYSTEM

Alcoholics frequently experience severe potassium loss. As most people will agree, drinking alcohol causes an increase in urination. With elimination, large mineral stores are depleted—zinc, potassium and magnesium to name just a few. These minerals are important to the maintenance of fluid balance and necessary for many chemical reactions in the body cells. More times than not, the alcoholic craves salt to replace potassium. This further reduces the potassium balance.

5

ALCOHOL ABUSE IN THE ELDERLY

ELDERLY ALCOHOLICS HAVE EI-
THER a forty or fifty year history of excessive drinking or a
moderate consumption which increases during times of stress.
This late alcohol abuse is often related to isolation, loneliness,
loss of spouse, illness and/or despair. This leads many to find
comfort in alcohol regardless of the consequences.

The effects of alcohol, at the cellular level, are altered due
to the physiological changes related to aging. The loss of lean
muscle mass may result in the reduction of alcohol distribution.
This results in increased concentration of ethanol. Therefore,
the amount of alcohol required to create dependency is considerably lower for the elderly. Most may be unaware their alcohol
consumption is affecting their health since quantities may be
relatively small. The elderly usually consume less alcohol than
the younger drinker to experience the same effect.

The Council of Scientific Affairs, American Medical Association cites the following findings that suggest problem drinking in older adults:

1 Cognitive decline or self-care deficit

2 Non-adherence with medical appointments

3 Recurrent accidents, injuries or falls

4 Frequent visits to the emergency room

5 Gastrointestinal disorder

6 Estrangement from family

7 Unexpected delirium during hospitalization

The symptoms of alcoholism in the elderly may go undetected for an extended period of time due to the variables of the aging process. Aging, for many, can be a time of diminished physical and psychological capacity. Any or all of the above symptoms may be experienced by the vast majority of the elderly. Whereas, in a younger patient, the findings would be linked to chronic alcoholism.

If a person were to stereotype an alcoholic as the obnoxious drinker, panhandler on the street or lush, those images somehow, would not apply to our senior citizens. For the most part, elderly alcoholics are quiet drinkers. They are rarely arrested for DUI, assault charges or family violence. In fact, they are usually the victim.

The effects of alcohol produce a pronounced response in the elderly who are on prescribed medication. Some of their drugs may interact with alcohol, producing further confusion and physical toxicity. Such alcohol/medication interaction can be dangerous or even fatal.

The following is a list of medical problems, in the elderly, adversely influenced by alcohol.

1 Hypertension

2 Ulcers

3 Gastrointestinal distress

4 Pancreatitis

5 Diabetes mellitus

6 Depression

7 Profound cerebral atrophy

In later years, age 70 and beyond, alcohol consumption appears to decline. Reasons for this decrease may include advanced medical problems, financial strain and few social gatherings.

The story that follows is Atypical of what happens to the majority of elderly who abuse alcohol.

LIONEL AGE 69

Lionel is a retired naval officer. He had never had any major medical problems or mental disorders. He has been drinking for many years and does not believe alcoholism is a disease. He refers to it as a lack of will power. He admits he has signs of alcohol dependency, but states, "I can quit anytime I want."

Lionel and his brother Fred took a cruise to St. Thomas, Virgin Islands. While at sea, Fred noticed Lionel spent most of his time in the cabin. When he did come out, it was for meals (he ate sparingly) and night life. Fred commented on his brother's behavior and personal appearance. Lionel's response: "I'm on vacation."

Fred and Lionel visited the port of St. Thomas, but Lionel

seemed more interested in the night life instead of touring.

When they arrived home, Fred confronted Lionel about his excessive drinking. Obviously, Fred had never noticed his brother's alcohol abuse before this time.

With some prompting from Fred, Lionel visited his family physician and intervention followed shortly. Lionel was fortunate. He wasn't on any medication, he had prompt intervention and family support.

Over time, alcohol dependence, without intervention will ravage the mind and body. The consequences can be devastating.

It is important for the physician to carefully review the prescription and over-the-counter medications being taken by the patient and adjust them accordingly. Careful evaluation of the physical and mental state is needed. A nutritional consultant may find the client physically fragile. Appropriate measures should be taken to bring the patient/client to a state of well-being.

6

HYPOGLYCEMIA
AND ALCOHOLISM

To a greater or lesser degree, all alcoholics suffer from biochemical imbalance. They eat poorly and in the advanced stage of alcoholism malnutrition exists. The major portion of calories comes from the alcohol itself. This leads to depletion of essential vitamins and minerals. Without sufficient amounts of thiamine, niacin, folic acid, potassium, calcium, magnesium, B12 and the essential amino acids, the alcoholic does not have the resources to create bone, red blood cells or health body tissue.

With increased alcohol consumption there is loss of appetite. Direct exposure to ethanol damages the gastric mucosal barrier. This membrane is composed of cells which secrete various forms of mucus in the lining of the gastrointestinal tract.

During the advanced stage, alcoholics are generally in such a weakened condition they neither have the desire nor the ability to eat. This only compounds the seriousness of the existing nutritional deficiencies. Depletion of the B vitamins plagues the alcoholic. Irritability is experienced, loss of mental clarity, fatigue and emotional instability. These physiological and psychological problems are also encountered in the early stages.

Faulty body chemistry shows up on the glucose tolerance test. The majority of alcoholics have hypoglycemia (low blood sugar). This is a disturbance in sugar metabolism. It is an abnormally diminished content of glucose in the blood accompanied by headache, confusion, hallucinations and has even been known to result in convulsions and coma.

Broad swings in blood glucose seriously impair physical and emotional stability. The multiple nutrient deficiencies created by alcohol abuse have been reversed following the ingestion of wholesome foods and therapeutic amounts of vitamins and minerals.

Vitamin and mineral supplementation is essential. However, they are not to be taken in place of good food, but in addition to nutritious meals. The importance of proper diet cannot be overemphasized. The diet should include whole grains, plenty of fresh vegetables and some fruit. Sugar and white flour products should be avoided as much as possible. Through a sound nutritional approach, it is easier for the alcoholic to remain sober.

Years of deficiencies need to be made up. It can be ascertained that protein foods (lean meats, fish, legumes with brown rice) are particularly required. Stabilizing blood sugar enables other treatments to be more effective.

In 1975, Dr. Ross noted three stages to the hypoglycemic condition:

Stage 1—The patient experiences an increased craving for sweets and starchy foods. Depression appears and can be so severe as to require antidepressant medication, and occasionally admission to the hospital.

Stage 2—Patients suffer from recurrent episodes of their typical hypoglycemic symptoms, interposed with episodes of well-being.

Stage 3—Constant, almost persistent symptoms are experienced. It is almost impossible to counter the drive for junk food.

Progress is made once the alcoholic identifies their problem and associates it with junk food. Dr. Ross stated, "If a relapse occurs, one should investigate the diet to determine how this could have developed. When this is found and eliminated, the patient will recover." This theory holds true to this day.

In November 2000, Dr. David Overstreet, an associate professor of psychiatry stated, "Several years ago, we found clinical evidence linking a liking for sweets with alcoholism in a study that involved subjects tasting a wide range of concentrations of table sugar in water."

Sweets are usually craved when nervous or depressed. Most alcoholics believe eating sweets makes them feel better. But, when the blood sugar level drops fatigue, irritability, depression and hyper-emotional states set in. The list of hypoglycemia symptoms is quite long and includes mental, physical and emotional etiology.

The brain is one part of the body that has a specific need for a constant glucose supply. When the pancreas over produces insulin and the blood sugar level falls dangerously low, the brain is deprived of essential nutrients and is literally starved. It cannot develop the energy to feed its' cells from fats and protein. If hypoglycemia is severe and prolonged, permanent brain damage can occur.

Most alcoholics supply themselves with empty calories. Even on their "road to recovery," whether in a hospital, rehabilitation center, or at an Alcoholics Anonymous meeting, the "yo-yo syndrome" (rising and falling blood sugar) continues. It is at these very places where the alcoholic can get all the coffee and pastry his or her heart desires. The coffee is constantly being brewed, while the sugary confections are ever present for the taking.

Chronic low blood sugar levels create psychosomatic (mental and physical) illness. The brain is not the only area of involvement. There is a body-mind connection.

Neurological—Headache, tremor, dizziness, crying spells, insomnia and phobias

Physical—Sweating, rapid heartbeat and chronic indigestion.

We know alcoholism is a progressive, degenerative disease. Coupled with hypoglycemia, the results can be devastating. Let's examine like symptoms occurring from alcohol abuse and low blood sugar. Dizziness is found among those abusing alcohol; conversely, dizziness appears regularly among those with low blood sugar. Alcoholics have been known to experience multiple headaches within one days time. These symptoms typify hypoglycemia. Hypnogogic hallucination is another classic symptom. The hypnogogic state is that time just prior to sleep. Both low blood sugar and alcohol abuse can cause pathological drowsiness and false perception. Muscle cramps are a frequent annoyance, as is restless leg syndrome. The latter condition is characterized by an irritating sensation deep inside the leg muscles. Relief comes from constant leg movement. Edema (fluid retention) takes place in a high percentage of alcoholics and hypoglycemics. It is fair to say the symptoms of alcohol abuse can be reproduced on a continual basis, even after sobriety, as long as the alcoholic is involved with high doses of sugar and hydrolyzed starch foods. Nutritional education is important for everyone, since we are all vulnerable to disease.

In 1989, a group of Peruvian peasants were studied. They showed symptoms of mental disease from poor nutrition. Dr. R. Bolton states:

"They fought amongst themselves, had a high incidence of theft, rape, homicide and divorce. Out of 1,200 men, half of them were involved in homicide. The probable reason for this dilemma: consuming lots of alcohol and chewing cola. Half of the population, when treated, was found to be hypoglycemic. Their aggressiveness and irritability assuredly came via improper nutrition."

Hypoglycemia is prevalent in the United States, not just among alcoholics, but the public in general. Our diets are generally poor, consisting mainly of refined carbohydrates, fast food and processed foods. People's addictions are being fed. Nutrients essential to good health and well-being are lacking in most diets.

Over the past thirty five years, our consumption of sugar has increased more than 35%. The average person eats approximately two pounds of sugar per week. Some people consume more, some slightly less. Much of this sugar is hidden. It is added, with great zeal, to baked goods and snacks.

Alcoholism and hypoglycemia not only cause the often mentioned physical and neurological symptoms, but the outer being suffers as well. The skin and hair are dry and itchy. The complexion is very often pasty in appearance, taking on a grayish tone. The eyes are dull, lacking sparkle and shine. Biochemical rebalancing will alter these disturbances.

While reviewing some ancient literature, the author came upon a book which takes an in depth look at the relationship between hypoglycemia and alcoholism. This work, researched by C. Jean Poulos, et.al., demonstrated and proved that alcoholism causes hypoglycemia. The research team also felt that hypoglycemia contributed to the problem of alcoholism.

The schizophrenic/ alcoholic has marked perceptual distortions. When the clinical syndrome of hypoglycemia exists, you have one of the most common causes of neurophychiatric illness.

The correction of this blood sugar disorder can save alcoholics years of agony. Extraordinary improvement and recovery has been made by persons receiving proper nutritional counseling.

IS HYPOGLYCEMIA A DISEASE

It has been duly noted in all existing literature that hypoglycemia *is not* a disease. Dorland's medical dictionary defines the word disease as:

"Any deviation from or interruption of the normal structure of function of any part, organ or system (or combination thereof) of the body that is manifested by a characteristic set of symptoms and signs and whose etiology, pathology and prognosis, may be known or unknown."

For hundreds of years the dis-ease of the alcoholic was looked upon as a public obscenity and family nuisance. Finally, the medical profession proclaimed it to be a disease. Today, another disease exists which is being passed over. The disruptive, often irritable, ill individual who is experiencing the dis-ease of hypoglycemia is not being taken seriously. Thousands of people are suffering needlessly. Doctors need to give their patients the six-hour glucose tolerance test and not the usual three hour test. The last three hours are crucial. It is in those final hours a person can be determined whether or not he/she is borderline or falls within the range for diagnoses. The author may stand alone in her belief, hypoglycemia is a disease, as is alcoholism. However, since hypoglycemia is in its' infancy, it will be some time before it is recognized for what it truly is, a family member to alcoholism. Detection and treatment of alcoholism and hypoglycemia are a positive step in preventative medicine.

A LIFETIME OF SABOTAGE

Is there anyone out there who would be harmed by improving their diet? Ignoring physical, mental and emotional problems will not make them go away. Alcoholism and hypoglycemia will not disappear by pretending they do not exist. People are the end result of their nutrition, behavioral training, and relationships. No one experiences one particular set of symptoms for alcoholism or hypoglycemia. As previously stated, "Stress takes its' toll on every individual, but the effects may be different." This is one of the reasons men and women who abuse alcohol often cannot recognize their problem. It is believed, by some, if you do not require hospitalization or are not falling down drunk, then there is no problem regardless of how many other dilemmas are present.

Homeostasis is the tendency to stability in the normal body states (internal environment) of the organism. When the pancreas sends out too much insulin, causing a rapid fall in blood sugar, the adrenal glands are called upon to do their job. Epinephrine, the hormone of the adrenal medulla, is released to assist in restoring blood sugar levels to normal. Now sugary delights are placing an added burden on the adrenal glands as well. People spend a lifetime sabotaging themselves and call it living.

Alcoholics usually range between periods of sobriety and intoxication. It is during this sober time when most have a craving for sweets. Ice cream, cakes, donuts, candy, cookies and an array of other sweets are desired. This craving calls for a glucose tolerance test.

Abstinence from alcohol is not the key to all the answers. Abnormal metabolic processes must be corrected.

Programs have been developed to follow-up the successful cases (those receiving nutritional therapy, A.A. and counseling), but what happens to the individual who starts a program and doesn't follow through?

TOM AGE 47

Tom's life is not unlike that of many alcoholics. His wife Norma goes on to say:

"Tom was raised in a one parent home with seven other siblings and an alcoholic mother. At the age of five, Tom was removed from the home, along with the other children, and placed in various orphanages. Since the family was scattered, Tom was alone. He spent the next twelve years of his life in a series of foster homes. At seventeen, his oldest sister signed him into the navy. I met Tom when he came home from boot camp. After a little while we started going out and Tom began what he called "partying." After eight months we got married and wound up having five kids. Tom's partying wasn't often, but when he did drink, it was a lot. We separated often only to get back together to start fresh. By 2002, his drinking was out of control. He was hospitalized for three weeks and said the fear of God was in him.

He experienced D.T.'s, edema and a swollen liver."

During the past two years, Tom has been consistently incon-sistent with his diet. If his wife hands him his dinner and food supplements, Tom will adhere to the program. For the past five months, Norma had decided to make Tom responsible for his own health and well-being. Their life together has once again be-come a nightmare. His diet is based on coffee (8 to 10 cups daily), cigarettes (2 packs a day) and basically sweets and deep fried foods. He has been attending A.A. meetings hoping to stay sober.

Tom is experiencing confusion, mood swings, depression, emotional and physical withdrawal from his family. This be-havior may result in Tom picking up a drink. We hope not.

Tom is like so many others out there. He could very easily be put on prescription medication. This would not be a positive influence on his life. A restricted nutritional program produces remarkable results. How can the human brain, which is being deprived of vital nutrients on a daily basis, be expected to make rational decisions? It is the contention of many Americans that medication, hospitals and rehabilitation centers sole purpose is to rescue those who abuse themselves. Such is not the case. All of the facilities and drugs combined cannot be all things to all people. It is each individuals responsibility to take care of their own health when given the appropriate tools to do so.

ALCOHOLISM AND ALLERGIES

Hypoglycemia is almost invariably found with alcohol abuse. Whether the alcohol addiction precedes or antecedes the hypo-glycemia, it is made worse by the use of alcohol.

Refined sugar products are abused by the alcoholic. They provide quick energy for the individual with low blood sugar level. However, the abuse of sugar and alcohol alone may not be the ensuing cause of low blood sugar.

Allergic reactions to certain foods other than sugar may also lower blood sugar. It is also possible that allergies other than food allergies may also cause blood sugar levels to plummet. A low blood sugar level tends to aggravate allergic reactions thus causing the patient to become enmeshed in a vicious cycle.

The author suggests that no patient with hypoglycemia can be properly treated without an allergy workup. Many people with hypoglycemia also have food allergies.

Since alcohol is made from some of the most common allergens—wheat, corn, yeast and sugar, focus should be placed on allergens and alcohol. The possibility exists that the alcoholic would be unaware of their allergy. Rather than experience a totally negative reaction, the alcoholic feels uplifted, relaxed, happy. Later, undesirable ramifications arise in the form of headache, irritability and/or gastric problems. As the disease progresses, rather than go through withdrawal from the alcohol, craving for the substance causes the allergic individual to take repeated doses to delay any negative reactions. There is convincing correlation between allergy and alcoholism.

Alcohol metabolizes quickly and creates an excessive influx of sugar. When alcohol is combined with an allergen, the combination forces the blood sugar down even more quickly.

Since the alcoholic generally eats poorly and is likely to be malnourished, they are a likely candidate for hypoglycemia and/or allergies. Poor nutrition lowers the body's immune system, leading to allergic reactions. It is vital to determine whether hypoglycemia and/or allergies are playing a role in the alcoholic's behavior. If this is the case, all of the psychotherapy in the world, individual or group, will not alter the cravings or behavior.

If the alcoholic follows the hypoglycemic diet and still experiences adverse symptoms, there is a possibility a food is triggering the reaction and needs to be removed from the diet. There are various ways to determine food allergies. An allergist may perform a skin or scratch test. However it is safe to say they are only about 20% accurate. The sublingual test is far more accurate. A diluted solution of the suspected offender is placed under the tongue. Absorption into the bloodstream is more rapid this way and the central nervous system reacts rather than just the skin. The entire system can be observed, both mental and physical. Then there is the pulse test. Upon waking, take your pulse before getting out of bed. Take the pulse again after being up and about for a few minutes. Add the two numbers, then divide by two. You now have what is called your mean pulse rate. Ten minutes after your meal, take your pulse. If the pulse rate increases by as little as ten points, one of the foods eaten may be an allergen.

No significant research has been done on the effect of allergies on alcoholism. Allergies are now appearing to be the root cause of much mental and physical illness. The fact that allergies may play a role in alcoholism should not be ignored.

Supplements that help build the immune system are of first importance. Both vitamin C and pantothenic acid are powerful agents for the immune system and improved adrenal function. Pyridoxine (B6) is needed for the production of antibodies.

It is important for the health care provider to explore all possibilities for the alcoholic seeking relief.

7

PHARMACOLOGIC TREATMENT

Alcoholism places a consid-
erable economic burden on society. Each year, an estimated
100,000 people die from alcohol related causes and 185 billion
dollars is spent yearly on direct or indirect health costs.

The focus of this chapter is to determine which pharmacologic treatments are most likely to enable alcoholics to achieve
long-term sobriety.

As established, people with the disease of alcoholism experience a host of symptoms. To differentiate between the complications of the illness itself and the side effects of prescription drugs
is a difficult task. An alcoholic may be taking an antidepressant
for a period of time feeling that he/she is either staying the same
or perhaps, feeling worse. The symptoms they are experiencing
may de due, in part, to the side effects of their medication.

The first few days of medication may find the patient with

excessive thirst, mild nausea and diarrhea. Not recognizing these signs as side effects to their medication, some out-patients have been known to take it upon themselves to increase the dosage, hoping to improve their dis-ease. The nausea and diarrhea worsen and the patient becomes confused and depressed.

The side effects of many prescription drugs are drowsiness, fatigue and lack of muscle coordination, to name a few. Some medications may be physically and psychologically habit-forming. It is the physicians responsibility to make their patient aware of the implications.

Abrupt discontinuation, of some medications, after taking them for a period of time, can cause convulsion, tremor, vomiting and sweating. None of the aforementioned conditions are desirable for anyone, much less the alcoholic who is trying to reconstruct his/her life.

The following story expresses the dilemma related to alcohol abuse and the side effects of medication. John entered the hospital hoping to get relief from his already tortured body, only to give the following account:

JOHN AGE 43

"My doctor prescribed Nefazodone, an antidepressant. I believed it would relieve my depression, increase my physical activity, improve my appetite and help me sleep. I was not aware of the side effects of the medication. There were changes in my heart rate and I experienced anxiety. If that wasn't enough, I also had a case of constipation. Later, I found myself taking medication to counteract the side effects of the Nefazodone. Soon after, I was vomiting and had diarrhea. I became confused as to whether the symptoms were coming from my alcohol withdrawal or coming from the drugs."

These are just some of the adverse side effects. John went on to experience more. One drug would produce negative symptoms, while two (that were contraindicated) would worsen matters. Since all of the side effects mirrored John's drinking disorder, there was confusion concerning further treatment of his illness.

Studies have been made comparing a variety of drugs with placebo. The purpose of the studies was to evaluate outcomes of abstinence, treatment, compliance and medication side effects.

MEDICATIONS EFFECT ON ALCOHOLISM

Before prescribing medication, the physician should consider the cumulative and synergistic effect it will have on the patient.

The following is a list of drugs currently being used to treat alcoholism, their effect and side effect.

ACAMPROSATE

This medication has increased the number of non-drinking days by 50%. There is a higher abstinence rate and less severe relapse. Treatment is positive when applied in a community-based rehabilitation program. Side effect: diarrhea.

DISULFIRAM

This drug provides moderate reduction in drinking. However, there is no improvement in abstinence. Disulfiram should never be taken with alcohol. Side effect: diarrhea, headache, nausea and dizziness.

LITHIUM

Prescribed for manic depression, it appears to be non-effective in abstinence. Side effect: nausea, diarrhea, vomiting, drowsiness, confusion, abdominal pain and lack of coordination.

NALMEFENE

Helps reduce heavy drinking. Similar to Naltrexon. Side effect: acceptable, less toxic to the liver.

NALTREXON

This medication is approved by the FDA for alcohol dependence. It helps reduce drinking, but only in combination with psychotherapy. The success of this drug may come from the blockage of pleasure produced by alcohol. Side effect: Significant nausea, joint pain, abdominal cramps, headache, dizziness, insomnia, vomiting, depression and diarrhea. When taken in excessive doses, it has been known to cause hepatitis or liver failure.

Of the aforementioned drugs, Acamprosate appears to be a well-tolerated pharmacologic adjunct to psychosocial and nutritional treatment of alcoholism.

All results of taking the previously named medication are pursuant to the patients compliance with treatment. For those patients who do not adhere to their program, relapse rates will be high.

The administration of prescription drugs has been addressed by the Physicians Guide to Helping Patients with Alcohol Problems. It was released in 1995 by the National Institute on Alcohol Abuse and Alcoholism. It is a step by step approach in identifying alcohol problems. It is based on more than twenty years of research on alcohols effect on health.

The Physicians Guide enables physicians to evaluate high and low risk drinkers.

According to Richard Fuller, M.D., director of NIAAA's Division of Clinical and Prevention Research:

"Brief interventions to reduce alcohol consumption should be conducted by or under the supervision of a health professional.

Patients who attempt to reduce their drinking should continue to be professionally evaluated and monitored."

HOSPITALIZATION FOR ALCOHOLISM

If the disease of alcoholism is detected early, outpatient treatment is viable. When severe metabolic abnormality exists, from uncontrollable drinking, an inpatient setting is necessary. This would assure adequate hydration and monitoring of medical conditions.

Within 10 to 72 hours, the state of alcohol withdrawal occurs. This is due to abstaining, after chronic ingestion. The symptoms can range from mild to severe. Anxiety, confusion, shakiness and sweating spells are experienced. In severe cases, delirium tremens (D.T.s) result. This is all due to nervous system toxicity. At this time medication is prescribed to ease the symptoms of withdrawal and relieve the craving for alcohol.

The hospitals approach to the alcoholic is behavioral. The intensity of the approach varies from hospital to hospital. Individual and/or group counseling is provided in many hospitals.

There are many patients who are adamant about ingesting food. These patients should be given liquid drinks (Ensure) as they contain a wide range of vitamins and minerals, and is easily digested. The intestinal tract, at this time, requires gentle stimulation. After long periods of alcohol abuse, the body will rely on its' own tissue for nourishment. During this process, the intestinal wall becomes extremely thin.

HOSPITALIZATION AND THE ELDERLY

Alcohol related hospitalization of the elderly is common in the United States.

Most elderly alcoholics drink to cope with life, not to become intoxicated. No longer feeling safe, secure and in control, they reach for the alcohol to temporarily lessen their anxiety.

When they are admitted into the hospital, scheduling treatment becomes difficult. The diagnostic tools commonly used for alcoholism are not well suited to the elderly since many have dementia. Once protocol has been established, alcohol withdrawal in the elderly must be closely supervised. Treatment of elderly alcoholics requires great skill, sensitivity and respect by all health care providers.

Upon discharge, a frail elderly alcoholic may benefit from referral to an appropriate agency for home care or Nursing home placement. The latter would be appropriate for long-term alcoholics with physical problems and/or dementia.

Although some treatment programs appear to help the alcoholic, there is still considerable relapse. The author has reason to believe that proper nutrition offers an effective adjunct therapy to the treatment of alcoholism.

8

A SELF-HELP GROUP AND
SUCCESS RATING

"WHENEVER ANYONE, ANYWHERE, REACHES out for help, I want the hand of A.A. always to be there. For that, I am responsible." Bill Wilson.

When Bill W. and Dr. Bob founded Alcoholics Anonymous in 1935, alcoholism was not accepted as a disease by society or the medical profession. It wasn't until five years later that the medical community recognized alcoholism for what it was: a progressive, debilitating disease.

Since then, self-help groups have evolved throughout the United Stated. Each group focuses on a particular family member: (Alateen) for the youth of America, (Alanon) for the non-drinker, (ACOA) adult children of alcoholics and the father of them all, Alcoholics Anonymous.

One of America's greatest health problems has the distinction of being turned over to Alcoholics Anonymous by doctors, social workers and family counselors. Alcoholics Anonymous is a spiritual program consisting of twelve steps. The "road to recovery" is experienced by those who are willing to take the first step: "We admitted we were powerless over alcohol, that our lives had become unmanageable." For most alcoholics, this is a difficult task. A.A. members list less that 42% of all alcoholics in the United States.

The twelve step guide that follows has been the foundation and motivating force for other self-help groups.

TWELVE STEP GUIDE

1 We admitted we were powerless over alcohol—that our lives had become unmanageable.

2 Came to believe that a Power greater than ourselves could restore us to sanity.

3 Made a decision to turn our will and our lives over to the care of God, as we understood Him.

4 Made a searching and fearless moral inventory of ourselves.

5 Admitted to God, to ourselves, and to another human the exact nature of our wrongs.

6 Were entirely ready to have God remove all these defects of character.

7 Humbly asked Him to remove our shortcomings.

8 Made a list of all persons we had harmed, and became willing to make amends to them all.

9 Made direct amends to such people wherever possible, except

when to do so would injure them or others.

10 Continued to take personal inventory and when we were wrong promptly admitted it.

11 Sought through prayer and meditation to improve our conscious contact with God as we understood Him, praying only for knowledge of His will for us and the power to carry that out.

12 Having had a spiritual awakening as the result of these steps, we tried to carry this message to alcoholics, and to practice these principles in all our affairs.

This twelve step program has enabled thousands of men and women to refrain from using alcohol for extended periods of time and for some, permanently. Alcoholics Anonymous "Easy Does It," "One Day At A Time" approach encourages alcoholics to reduce stress and live in the moment.

Alcoholics Anonymous offers emotional support, anonymity and confidentiality and the discovery that the alcoholic is not alone with their disease. Members are encouraged to share their feelings on how the alcohol has affected them. These experiences are shared as a means to ventilate and also to be of assistance to other people in a similar situation. Alcoholics and therapists alike believe these meetings provide insight into the drinking disorder and how it effects others. It gives alcoholics an opportunity to meet people from all walks of life, to witness them in various stages of recovery, and motivates each one to become more responsible for their own recovery process.

In order for the afflicted party to enter into a recovery phase, discussion of personal conflicts and inadequacy is important. Alcoholics Anonymous is crucial to behavior modification.

Regarding the success rate of treatment: available statistics showing the success rate is subject to criticism. What is success? The author has defined success by observing, "Not where the person is today, but how far they have come to get here." To once again function within the family unit, to hold down a job, attend school on a regular basis and have regained self-confidence and self-respect should be taken into consideration when determining the success rate of *any* program. If success will only be defined by the length of time the alcoholic abstains, then there is no program that will be deemed successful. Observations of any program depend on one's interpretation of success.

Most everyone afflicted has reverted to their destructive drinking behavior, no matter how temporary. In fact, it is fairly common for the alcoholic to relapse upon discharge from the hospital. The thought of every day living, for some alcoholics, becomes overwhelming. When behavior becomes self-destructive and life threatening, the issue is critical. When that same individual can go for a period of time (several months to several years) diminishing destructive behavior and increasing the constructive, he/she can be considered successful.

Bill W. extolled the virtues of niacin (B3), pyridoxine (B6), and ascorbic acid (vitamin C) along with a protein diet in the control of alcoholism. He attributed this nutritional routine as the major factor in his own control over the disease. This led him to print a booklet about the advantages of vitamin therapy in the control of alcoholism.

9

THE ROAD BACK—A WHOLE FOODS APPROACH

"WE ADMITTED WE WERE powerless over alcohol, that our life had become unmanageable." With the help of a Greater Power, the alcoholic attends their first A.A. meeting. The men and women, at the meeting, are open and friendly. They attempt to make the new comer feel welcome and comfortable. The alcoholic sits and listens to the guest speaker. The story being told is astounding. The new comer begins to second guess. What am I doing in this place? He/she cannot relate to the speaker. After all, the visitor hasn't done half the things being discussed. This speaker has a real problem, not me. The new comer leaves the meeting and goes to the nearest bar, or perhaps waits one day and then indulges. The alcohol lessens their anxiety and frees their inhibitions.

With this unrealistic glimpse of reality, they temporarily become the person they would like to be. The vicious cycle begins. The road back is never easy.

Alcohol goes back to primitive man who believed this was a gift from the gods, and so it was called spirits. With that in mind, some people think drinking alcohol makes them more socially acceptable.

Alcohol burns in the body as a food. One ounce of alcohol contains 210 calories. However, no one can exist on alcohol alone. Prolonged periods of drinking alcohol depletes the vitamin B complex in the body.

DEFICIENCY SIGNS OF B COMPLEX

Heart palpitation
Ache all over feeling
Sore tongue
Abnormally tired
Diastolic blood pressure over 90
Many vague fears
Feel others are against you
Hands and/or feet tingle
Forgetful
Confused about life and your purpose in it.

Experiencing any or all of the above symptoms, the alcoholic drinks all the more, not to run away from life, but to find it. In the early stages, life appears to become more abundant through the use of alcohol. Problems appear to be resolved. Unfortunately, over time, the quantity must be increased to produce the desired effect. The following is an account given to the author by her client.

TONY AGE 27

"My first A.A. meeting didn't work for me, but I went to another one because I smashed up the car the other night and to get my wife off my back, I decided to give it another try. As I was sitting there listening to some "guy with a problem" speak, my gut started killing me. My appetite isn't what it used to be, and I guess my alcohol, at times, has become my lunch and dinner. I really wanted to get out of that place (the meeting). Then I go home and listen to my wife complain. I feel like my nerves are screaming. She claims our sex life doesn't exist. We used to have plenty, but I'm tired. How could anyone feel good and get a decent nights sleep living with her."

Tony's entire being is crying out for help. After attending the meeting, he wondered how he would ever make it without another drink.

One part of Tony's story brings up the next topic:

ALCOHOL AND SEX

One area that has not been discussed is sexual problems. The following is a frequent complaint: "My wife, husband, lover doesn't turn me on anymore." Many of the foods being neglected by the alcoholic are excellent sources of vitamins, minerals, necessary fatty acids and essential amino acids necessary for proper functioning of the sex glands. The male sex gland cannot perform properly without zinc and manganese. Vitamin E has been lauded as a sexual enhancer since it has circulation-stimulating properties. It increases cardiac efficiency and stamina. Male impotence is often likely to be the result of hypoglycemia. At the Tel Aviv Medical School in Israel, doctors researched abnormal carbohydrate metabolism and found that it contributed to male impotence at all ages.

Low sex drive disrupts many relationships and can be traced directly to overall nutritional deficiencies. Sexual activity, or lack thereof, is an easily disturbed body function. This is one of the common complaints of the alcoholic.

THE CHEMICAL CUISINE

The book, thus far, has given insight regarding alcohol abuse. Stories have been introduced excerpting the lives of alcoholics regardless of age, gender or race. You have discovered that alcoholism has no boundaries. It afflicts the affluent as well as the needy. With this information in mind, it is time to move on.

The ultimate goal of this book is to provide each reader with the tools necessary for building their highest level of health and encouragement to use the knowledge. We know the cause and effects of the alcoholic's health problems and only in the role of teacher can the nutritional consultant help the alcoholic understand how their food choices are effecting their health and assist them in finding solutions.

In addition to being physically stressed through malnourishment, the alcoholic is in a state of great mental and emotional anguish. The very best of foods are required during this time of crisis. However, sound nutrition involves more than an allotted number of calories, divided amongst the four basic food groups.

Over the past two decades, countless articles and books on health and nutrition have been written. Each has given a different point of view on the subject. Some of the new techniques have been met with controversy by the Scientific Community at the time of their presentation.

It has been suggested that we eat all raw food and that our

fruit be consumed only in the morning. Should we all be veg-
etarians? Others say the key to good health is a high protein
low carbohydrate diet. So many choices, so much confusion.
Due to biochemical individuality, there is no one way for everyone to eat. The optimum food and supplemental program is
highly individualized. It requires time and experimentation to
come up with the best program for the individual need. Who
will decide whether the nutritional approach to the treatment
of alcoholism is worthy? If time is taken to listen to the body,
you can make that determination. The body will speak to you
of its' health or dis-ease.

While there is no panacea diet, there are basics to a diet
that provides healing from within and without. We hear a great
deal about whole foods, but what are they? The term whole
food, as used herein, refers to unadulterated, unprocessed, lacking additives and preservatives. Our food is being bombarded
with chemicals. Crops are sprayed with pesticides and grown
in denatured soil with chemical fertilizers causing many people
discomfort. The list of suspected carcinogenic additives, preservatives and dyes is in the thousands.

Why all this fuss over whole, natural food? Ingesting denatured food makes it difficult to regain and maintain wholistic
health. Whole foods are natural medicine for the body. Many
disorders can be ameliorated by selecting foods wisely.

Good health is not necessarily obtained solely through abstinence from alcohol or a new miracle drug. There is, however, evidence that the biochemical elements of sound nutrition
accelerates the healing/reversal process of treating alcoholism.
Sound nutrition is safe, effective and economical too.

When moving forward, the decision to choose optimal

health should be that of the alcoholic. Turning from alcohol abuse to a life of mental clarity, emotional stability and a sense of well-being calls for courage to withstand ridicule from peers. It requires the willingness to do the work, the determination to persevere and the vision to recognize potential.

We've all, at some point in our lives, witnessed people who appear to be fairly intelligent. The proper clothes are worn for the season of the year, the home is maintained to keep out excessive heat and cold and they are knowledgeable on the job. But, above all, they maintain their vehicle. It provides the transportation. It takes them where they want to go. Observe these same people, on the run, as they have coffee for breakfast. If time permits, they will include some type of pastry, stop for a double cheeseburger and fries for lunch and have a quick denatured meal for dinner. Most alcoholics sustain life in this fashion, but at what cost? Alcohol abuse + poor eating habits = poor health.

In the United States, the average person consumes approximately 125 pounds of sugar per year, 240 pounds of meat (that includes chicken and turkey) and only 10 pounds of whole grain. It then becomes easy to see the effect of such a diet not only on the body, but on the behavior as well. Extremes in eating and drinking result in extreme behavior. The person suffering from alcohol abuse experiences a lack of order and direction in their life. They are anxious, confused and stressed. The behavioral tendency on whole foods is more relaxed, active and alive.

Alcoholics need to know that the Standard American Diet (SAD) of hot dogs, hamburgers, fried foods, soft drinks and sugary delights is an invitation to misery.

In examining the foods most often consumed by alcoholics, refined carbohydrates and fried foods are on the top of the list.

Salty snacks such as potato chips, pretzels and corn chips place a close second. These foods are high in fat, sugar and sodium. Between the alcohol abuse and the nutritionally depleted diet, the gastrointestinal tract suffers and disorders are experienced. Gastritis (inflammation of the stomach), bloating, belching, gas, abdominal cramps, constipation and diarrhea are some of the symptoms which develop over time.

The gastrointestinal (GI) tract begins in the mouth and goes through to the anus. Digestion begins when food enters the mouth and mixes with saliva. The food then passes through the esophagus into the stomach where it is further broken down by digestive enzymes from the pancreas, gallbladder and liver. Most of the food absorption takes place in the small intestine before being passed to the large intestine for excretion.

Proper digestion is a requirement for good health. Focusing on a whole foods diet will help correct disorders of the gastro-intestinal tract. The body is a wondrous creation which, when given the essential nutrients via whole foods and food supplements will repair and regenerate itself.

Alcohol abuse and malnutrition is also a primary cause of most conditions of the male genitourinary tract. A whole foods approach to health is essential to normal function. To heal prostate tissue alcohol, caffeine and spicy foods must be avoided.

Since vitamins C, E and the mineral zinc are the most prominent elements found in prostate tissue, they are necessary for the formation of seminal fluid and healing.

Every cell, tissue and organ responds from eating healthy foods. Strength is gained and cell structure rejuvenated. Poor quality foods delay the healing process and often times exacerbate symptoms. Nutritional factors are probably the most significant for predisposing 75% of the alcoholics physical and mental symptoms.

Knowing which foods are more nutritious and why is an important component in the recovery from alcoholism. The current challenge is to look to the proper diet and level of nutrients that will help maintain a high level of wellness. To discover one's personal biochemical needs may take time and experimentation. To reduce the length of time, guess work and possible frustration, a person can consult a dietary/nutritional consultant. They will help access and develop a program to meet his/her biochemical individuality.

A whole foods approach may sound a bit overwhelming, but in the course of a lifetime it is worth the effort. Each person who chooses this option is not merely addressing their symptoms, but bringing balance to their being.

IO

THE OPTIMAL NUTRITIONAL PROGRAM

In order to create the optimal nutritional program for the treatment of alcoholism, observations were made in the health-disease category. First, it was informative to note the dietary patterns associated with this disease. Second, it was equally helpful to analyze the deficiencies in conjunction with the longevity of the disease and consistency of same.

Once the alcoholic decides to get on track, detoxification should be encouraged. This is a major step in restoring health, as it helps rid the body of negative conditions. However, if the body is frail, they may want to wait. It takes considerable energy to go through a cleanse.

During detoxification, the body goes through three stages:

catabolism, stabilization and anabolism.

Stage 1—Catabolism

Emphasis is on elimination. If the quality of food going into the body is of higher quality than the cellular environment, the body will begin to perform its' house cleaning. The lower grade materials (tissues, cells, etc.) will be replaced by superior tissue. Hardened fecal matter is excreted along with broken down tissues and old cells. As the body is throwing off toxins, skin rash may occur. No cause for alarm for the skin is the largest organ of elimination and will become more active. The body will be discarding toxins rapidly and saving the alcoholic from more serious problems. This is all part of the healing process. Some weight loss may be experienced.

Stage 2—Stabilization

The weight generally remains the same during this period and elimination is in proportion to the amount of new tissue being built by good food.

Stage 3—Anabolism

This is the building stage. Weight may increase even if the caloric intake is low. New tissue is being formed faster, due to better food. When chronic abuse of alcohol stops, a let down occurs due to the slower action of the heart. During this building up period, energies are concentrated on the reconstruction of vital organs and glands, and some weakness may be experienced. In actuality, the body is becoming stronger. This is a crucial time and more rest and sleep is necessary.

The recovery period is a time of adjustment. Eventually a marked improvement in vitality will be felt. However, if the alcoholic continually rearranges their nutritional program to suit their desires, dis-ease will become apparent.

WATER

Drinking water will now be discussed briefly. Water is a life-giving substance. Since the body is composed of approximately 70% water, it is necessary for all building functions in the body. Water carries the nutrients from the ingested food into the cells. It aids in digestion, absorption and excretion. Dehydration causes mental sluggishness, weakness, tiredness and joint discomfort. Once water intake is adjusted the above symptoms are lessened considerably.

Signs of Inadequate Water Intake

1 Bubbles in the urine

2 Amber colored urine without taking food supplements

3 A fishy odor

Research is in progress and treatments are being worked with and refined. This is happening from a psycho-therapeutic end of treatment to the behavioral. Health care providers are aware of the loss of essential nutrients during the drinking process. Yet, little mention is made of nutritional treatment for alcoholism in medical journals. These lost nutrients are not supplied through the diets found in most hospitals or rehabilitation centers. The following is the dietary experience of a client.

DAVID AGE 45

"Having hit the bottom of the barrel, my family decided to bring me to a New York hospital where I signed myself in. The wife and kids thought this would rehabilitate me. I was relieved to see the dietician intercede and make all the selections for my meals. When I was admitted, I felt mentally unable to make those decisions. I was grateful to get a sound nights sleep, get off the alcohol and have three square meals a day. Breakfast usually consisted of eggs, bacon or sausage, white toast, cereal, juice, coffee and sometimes a piece of fruit. Lunch could be macaroni and cheese or meat, gravy, some kind of vegetable, bread and dessert (cake, pudding, ice cream). Dinner was pretty much the same as lunch, with a change of meat. There was a coffee urn in the lounge and you could drink as much of it as you saw fit, all day, every day. I got medication for diarrhea, depression and insomnia."

David's wife asked the author to visit him. While at the hospital, she was disappointed to see so much emphasis placed on the quantity of food rather than the quality.

Several dieticians were interviewed in the upper New York State area and the dialogue delivered by all was, "We serve a balanced diet." The dietician at Conifer Park Treatment Center for Alcohol and Chemical Dependency, Gleville, N.Y. was kind enough to give the author the menu for the month. It was reviewed diligently. After careful consideration, the observations follow: since dieticians are trained to work with weights and measures, one cannot fault the menu coming from that school of thought. All portions are measured precisely and there is variety. However, eight eggs are allowed weekly along with bacon, ham and sausage. A considerable amount of read meat is served, as are fried foods. A sweet is served with each meal and peanut butter, jelly and crackers are available throughout the day. Coffee (regular) accompanies each meal. There is also a coffee urn in the lounge where it is available all day. Not unlike the hospital where David stayed. The dietician did mention, "The coffee in the lounge is decaf."

Most patients lean heavily on refined sugar products and coffee. Some of the food ingested by the patients is not nutritious. When asked about the drink Ensure, one dietician stated, "We discourage it. We would prefer the patients eat solid food." Patients in weakened conditions should be monitored carefully. Too many calories in the way of solid food, too soon, can cause a considerable amount of discomfort to the patient who has existed on alcohol and little else.

Considering traditional dietary menus, whether weekly or monthly, they are a high fat, high cholesterol, high sugar diet. Granted, these menus far surpass the usual eating habits of the chronic alcoholic, but this book is not about just getting by. It's about nutritional education for the treatment of alcoholism, so a person has the tools necessary to make intelligent choices for their health. The author uses the following analogy. "Most schools of thought pay attention to the physical body without observing the mental and/or emotional and visa versa. " She likens this to giving a person a set of plans and an empty tool box, then sending them off to create something wonderful. "Through this book, the reader is being given the tools to work with, as well as the skill required to read the plans and the ability to put that knowledge to good use."

If a person is in rehabilitation, important information should be provided. This information should logically explain what happens within the organism while drinking, the symptoms they experience versus hypoglycemia symptoms, the whole foods approach, supplementation of vitamins and minerals and a shopping list similar to the one that follows. The shopping list eases the decisions required to select nutritious foods.

DIET PROGRAMS

For the Health of it

SHOPPING LIST

Beans: Black eyed peas, garbanzo (chick peas), lentils, lima, navy, pinto, red, black

Beverages: Apple juice, decaffeinated coffee and tea, herb tea, lemon juice, lime juice, passion fruit juice, pineapple juice, prune juice and white grape juice

Bread: Oat, pumpernickel, rye, sourdough

Cereal: Grape nuts, oatmeal, granola, oat squares

Crackers: breadsticks, matzo, melba toast, rice cakes, rice crackers

Dairy: Eggs, egg beaters, yogurt, milk, lactaid 100

Dressings: Apple cider vinegar and lemon, oil and vinegar, fat free dressings

Fruit: Apples, apricots, banana, all berries, cantaloupe, cherries, grapefruit, grapes, honeydew, kiwi, mango, nectarine, orange, papaya, peach, pear, pineapple, plums, tangerine, watermelon

High Protein: Chicken, fish, tofu, turkey, low-fat cheese

Pasta: Spinach, vegetable, no yolk noodles

Rice: Basmati, brown, jasmine, saffron

Seasoning: Add herbs and/or pepper to season salads, soups, any food

Vegetables: Fresh, if frozen read labels for sugar and sodium content

Snacks: Almonds, dried fruits, fresh fruit, popcorn, rice cakes with fruit spread

GUIDELINES FOR A NUTRIENT BALANCED DIET
(More food or Less—Depending on Current Weight)

The following menus have been designed from the shopping list. If eating away from home, the menus may be used as a source of reference to pick and choose the most desirable foods for sustained recovery and well-being.

WEIGHTS AND MEASURES = CALORIC VALUE

1 Beans, nuts, seeds, eggs, meat. One serving =
½ cup dry beans, lentils, etc.
2 eggs
4 Tbs. peanut butter
½ cup nuts, seeds
½ cup tuna fish
4 oz. lean meat/poultry
Calorie range = 140 for 2 eggs to 400 for peanut butter
Servings per day: 2 to 3

2 Tofu or dairy. One serving =
1 cup tofu, yogurt or milk
1½ oz. hard cheese
Calorie range = 75 calories for tofu to 165 for cheese
Servings per day: 2

3 Whole grains
  1 slice grain bread
  ½ cup cooked cereal
  ½ cup rice or pasta
  4 crackers or 1 pancake
  ¾ cup dry cereal
  Calories = 70
  Servings per day: 4 to 6

4 High Starch vegetables. One serving =
  ½ cup corn, potato, beets, carrots, yams, peas
  squash, or green beans
  Calories = 70
  Servings per day: 1 to 2

5 Other vegetables. One serving =
  1 cup broccoli, cabbage, greens, brussel sprouts
  1½ to 2 cups lettuce or spinach
  ½ cup green peppers
  1 tomato
  Calories = 40
  Servings per day: 2
  PROTEIN NEEDS ARE MET BY
  Tofu, peas, beans, protein drink, fish, chicken, turkey

6 Fruits. One serving =
  1 apple, peach, pear, banana, orange
  4 prunes
  Calories = 40
  Servings per day: 2

7 Fats and oils. One serving =
   1 Tbs. vegetable oil, butter or margarine
   Calories = 100
   Servings per day: 1

RECOMMENDED FRUITS

Fruit	Amount allowed in one serving
Apple	1 medium
Apricots, fresh	2 medium or 3 small
Blackberries	¾ cup
Blueberries	½ cup
Cantaloupe	½ if small
Cherries	15
Grapefruit	½
Grapes	10
Nectarine	1
Orange	1
Peach	1
Pineapple	½ cup
Plums	2 medium or 3 small
Raspberries	¾ cup
Strawberries	1 cup
Tangerine	1
Watermelon	1 slice

All of the above fruits should be eaten fresh. Although the sugar in fruit is natural, eating more than the recommended servings, at one time, will cause the blood sugar level to fluctuate.

PAULINE GRAY

SAMPLE MENUS FOR ONE WEEK

DAY 1

BREAKFAST   1 cup milk
¾ cup cooked cereal
2 poached or boiled eggs or egg beaters
1 slice bread
1 tsp. spread
beverage

LUNCH   1 cup or bowl of soup
sliced turkey or chicken
lettuce, tomato
2 slices bread
1 apple
beverage

DINNER   Broiled or baked meat or fish
1 baked potato
2 cups vegetables
crackers
beverage

DAY 2

BREAKFAST   1 cup dry cereal
¾ cup milk
½ grapefruit
1 slice bread
1 tsp. spread
beverage

LUNCH   1 cup or bowl vegetable soup
mixed bean salad
fish
1 slice bread
fruit
beverage

DINNER   meat/fish
1 baked yam
2 cups vegetables
1 cup milk
beverage

DAY 3

BREAKFAST   ½ grapefruit
¾ cup cereal
1 cup milk
beverage

LUNCH   water packed tuna fish
lettuce/tomato
2 slices bread
small green salad
1 piece fruit
1 cup milk
beverage

DINNER Flounder
1 cup rice
2 cups mixed vegetables
fruit
beverage

DAY 4

BREAKFAST ¾ cup oatmeal
½ cup milk
1 slice bread
1 tsp. spread
fruit
beverage

LUNCH 1 cup or bowl soup
cottage cheese with fruit or vegetables
crackers
beverage

DINNER meat/fish
2 cups vegetables
salad
baked potato
1 cup milk
beverage

DAY 5

BREAKFAST 1 cup rice
1/4 cup raisins
1 cup milk
1 slice bread
beverage

LUNCH 1 cup or bowl of soup
salad
1 slice bread
beverage

DINNER meat/fish
2 cups vegetables
1 baked potato
beverage

DAY 6

BREAKFAST 3/4 cup bran cereal
1/2 cup milk
2 poached or boiled eggs or egg beaters
fruit
beverage

LUNCH chicken salad
2 slices bread
sliced tomato, lettuce
small salad
beverage

DINNER pasta with sauce/meatballs (optional)
salad
bread
fruit
beverage

DAY 7

BREAKFAST pancakes/waffles (whole grain)
1 cup milk
fruit
beverage

LUNCH 1 cup or bowl soup
large salad
1 piece bread
beverage

DINNER meat/fish
1 cup rice
2 cups vegetables
crackers
beverage

It is suggested that pork be eliminated from the diet and beef be eaten sparingly. Small snacks are often suggested. These might be taken mid-morning and mid-afternoon. Although it isn't listed in the daily menu, two to four cups of vegetables should be consumed daily since they are high in nutrient value. Whenever possible, try for more.

Water is important. Eight glasses of water daily is advised.

MEATLESS MENU

Bread, Cereal, Pasta—8 Servings Daily
(total, not each)
  1 slice whole grain bread
  ½ cup cooked cereal or 1 cup dry cereal
  ½ cup rice or pasta

Vegetables—4 Servings Daily
  ½ cup cooked vegetables or 1 cup raw

Meat Substitute—2 to 3 Servings Daily
  ½ cup cooked beans
  4 oz. tofu
  10 almonds

Fruit
  2 pieces daily or as designated on foods list

Dairy or alternative—2 Servings Daily
  1 cup soy, lactaid 100, milk

Menu might look something like:

  BREAKFAST 4 oz. dry cereal or 1 cup cooked
        ½ cup milk of choice
        1 piece of fruit
        beverage

  MID AM almonds

LUNCH 2 cups vegetables or salad
4 oz. tofu
½ cup chick peas

MID PM 1 piece fruit

DINNER 2 cups raw vegetables or 1 cup cooked
1½ cups pasta or rice
1 slice whole grain bread
1 cup milk
beverage

Complete proteins are necessary to sustain life. Every muscle, tendon, ligament, organ, gland and body part is made up of protein.

When choosing from the meatless menu, combining the foods in the following manner will provide complete protein without the use of animal products (meat).

Vegetables combined with one of the following: Beans, cheese, nuts, rice, seeds, soy milk, tofu and whole grains.

As to the amount of food ingested, remember, these are guidelines. Hardy, robust people may need larger portions. However, this is an excellent starting point for nourishment and sustained blood sugar levels.

Many alcoholics show improvement within a matter of weeks. There are those who may take one to three months before considerable improvement is noticed. This depends on the persons constitution and the extent of damage to the organism.

It goes without saying, "Human nature prompts many individuals to ask when it will be possible for them to cheat on their diet program." Once the body, mind and emotion experiences healing, cravings for sweets are seldom experienced, sometimes never.

If the alcoholic chooses to binge on sweets, the sugar will react in the body the same as alcohol. They are then back to Russian Roulette. The alcoholic who makes wise food choices will feel healthy, and above all, enjoy his/her new found sense of well-being and inner peace.

11

VITAMINS AND MINERALS

AN INSURANCE POLICY ON YOUR HEALTH

THERE HAS BEEN SO much talk over the years about vitamins, but what exactly are they? Vitamins are organic food substances found in all living matter. They are absolutely necessary for growth and health. The difference between good health and poor health is determined by the amount of these substances in the system.

Vitamins fall into two categories: Fat-soluble and water-soluble. Vitamins A, D, E and K are fat soluble. They are stored in the body. Water soluble vitamins are lost through elimination.

Many people believe, if they start to eat better, their body will receive all the vitamins it requires. This is far from true. Alcoholism is so complex that the alcoholic's body is depleted of vitamins and minerals beyond their belief. Various drugs, alcoholic beverages, white sugar and smoking create multiple deficiencies. The alcoholic's emotional disturbances and digestive difficulty can also cause an added need for supplementation.

Along with vitamins, alcoholics should also incorporate minerals, healthy fats and proteins on a daily basis. If there is a great deal of inconsistency with any program, no matter how good it is, it won't work as it should.

When the alcoholic eats sensible meals and includes food supplements, it's like taking out an insurance policy on his/her health. They have nothing to lose and only a harvest of excellent health to reap.

Following is a list of vitamins and minerals and their specific value to the body.

VITAMIN A

DEFICIENCY SIGNS	Dry, itchy, scaly skin, night blindness, low resistance to infection, itchy eyes, dry brittle hair, loss of weight
THERAPEUTIC VALUE	Acts as an antioxidant helping to protect cells and enables the body to utilize protein. Prevents respiratory infection, stimulates proper growth, prevents bleeding gums, keeps skin moist, prevents night blindness
FOOD SOURCE	Red peppers, green and yellow vegetables and fruits, and fish oil
DESTRUCTION	Taking mineral oil, the inhalation of air pollutants and laxatives

VITAMIN BI (THIAMINE)

DEFICIENCY SIGNS	Nervousness, poor appetite, heart pains, nerve deterioration, cardiac failure, intestinal disorders and reduced efficiency of the brain
THERAPEUTIC VALUE	Prevents fatigue, stimulates appetite, aids in preventing heart failure, is used in the treatment of alcoholism and is essential to prevent nervous disorders
FOOD SOURCE	Brewer's yeast, wheat germ, soy, green vegetables, dried beans, brown rice, whole grains, poultry and peanuts
DESTRUCTION	Cooking food, stress, sugar, lactation and fever

VITAMIN B2 (RIBOFLAVIN)

DEFICIENCY SIGNS	Cracks and sores at the corners of the mouth, frequent occurrence of bloodshot eyes, lack of energy, purplish/red tongue, inflammation
THERAPEUTIC VALUE	Prevents mouth sores, fatigue, is used in the treatment of alcoholism, promotes healthy skin and aids in metabolism
FOOD SOURCE	Green leafy vegetables, brewer's yeast, wheat germ, beans, cheese, eggs, fish, milk, poultry and nuts

DESTRUCTION Oral contraceptives, cooking, alcoholic beverages and antibiotics

VITAMIN B3 (NIACIN)

DEFICIENCY SIGNS Diarrhea, skin rash, tongue sores, muscle weakness, hallucinations, irritability, depression, backaches, headaches and insomnia

THERAPEUTIC VALUE Lowers blood cholesterol level, is used in the treatment of alcoholism and schizophrenia, promotes healthy skin and increases stamina

FOOD SOURCE Brewer's yeast, wheat germ, nuts, fish, poultry, broccoli, carrots, cheese, eggs, milk, potatoes, tomatoes, whole grains

DESTRUCTION Alcoholic beverages, sugar consumption and antibiotics

VITAMIN B6 (PYRIDOXINE)

DEFICIENCY SIGNS Eczema, mouth sores, skin rash, ulcers, menstrual disorders, rheumatism and convulsions

THERAPEUTIC VALUE Aids in the treatment of acne, promotes healthy skin, relieves menstrual and menopausal symptoms, leg cramps and muscle pain. It is necessary for normal functioning of the gastrointestinal tract

FOOD SOURCE Brewer's yeast, wheat germ, nuts, fish, sunflower seeds, bananas, eggs, whole grains and vegetables

DESTRUCTION Heat from cooking, oral contraceptives and the use of hormones

VITAMIN B12 (CYANOCOBALAMIN)

DEFICIENCY SIGNS Anemia, nervousness, insomnia, digestive and gastrointestinal disorders

THERAPEUTIC VALUE Used in the treatment of pernicious anemia and mental health. It strengthens the nervous system, aids digestion and absorption of foods and promotes energy

FOOD SOURCE Milk, eggs, cheese, meat, seafood and tofu. B12 is not found in vegetables

DESTRUCTION Vegetarianism (provided all animal products are eliminated from the diet) and oral contraceptives

VITAMIN C

DEFICIENCY SIGNS Bruising easily, bleeding gums, weakness, shortness of breath, sallow complexion and susceptibility to infection

SOBER FOR THE HEALTH OF IT

THERAPEUTIC VALUE
Prevents scurvy, promotes bone and tooth growth, keeps blood vessels healthy, speeds wound healing, protects against blood clotting and bruising, enhances immunity and aids in iron absorption

FOOD SOURCE
Green vegetables, berries, citrus fruits, strawberries, tomatoes, onions and rose hip

DESTRUCTION
Alcohol, oral contraceptives, stress and cigarette smoking (25mg. of C destroyed for each cigarette smoked)

VITAMIN D

DEFICIENCY SIGNS
Rickets, malformed chest and muscle twitching

THERAPEUTIC VALUE
Prevents all the clinical signs above

FOOD SOURCE
Fish, milk, cod liver oil, egg yolk, sweet potatoes and oatmeal

DESTRUCTION
Insufficient exposure to sunlight

VITAMIN E

DEFICIENCY SIGNS
Poor circulation, slow tissue healing and premenstrual syndrome

THERAPEUTIC VALUE
It is an antioxidant, reduces scarring, improves circulation and is useful in treating PMS

FOOD SOURCE Whole grains, green leafy vegetables, beans, nuts, seeds, brown rice, eggs, milk, oatmeal, sweet potatoes and wheat germ

DESTRUCTION Avoidance of the above foods and taking the mineral iron at the same time

VITAMIN K

DEFICIENCY SIGNS Profuse bleeding

THERAPEUTIC VALUE Normal blood clotting and conversion of glucose into glycogen for storage in the liver

BIOTIN

DEFICIENCY SIGNS Lack of appetite, depression, muscular aches and pains, dull lifeless hair and skin

THERAPEUTIC VALUE Needed for the metabolism of fats, proteins and carbohydrates

FOOD SOURCE Peanuts, beans, eggs, whole grains, milk, poultry and yeast

DESTRUCTION Destroyed by a substance of raw egg white

CHOLINE

DEFICIENCY SIGNS High blood pressure, liver infections and cirrhosis of the liver

| THERAPEUTIC VALUE | Protects against fatty liver, helps manufacture thyroid hormones, keeps the nervous system healthy and is a treatment for viral hepatitis |

FOOD SOURCE — Whole grains, vegetables, egg yolks, beans, meat, milk, and whole grains

FOLIC ACID

DEFICIENCY SIGNS — Gastrointestinal problems, diarrhea, sore red tongue and pernicious anemia

THERAPEUTIC VALUE — Good for pregnant and lactating women. Protects against atherosclerosis, helps depression and anxiety

FOOD SOURCE — Green vegetables, brewer's yeast, beans, brown rice, chicken, milk, salmon, tuna and wheat germ

DESTRUCTION — Excessive demands on the body and metabolic derangement

INOSITOL

DEFICIENCY SIGNS — Fatty liver, high cholesterol and unhealthy hair

THERAPEUTIC VALUE — Removes fat from the liver, aids in cholesterol metabolism and helps with hair growth

FOOD SOURCE   All fruits, meat, milk, vegetables and whole grains

DESTRUCTION   Heavy caffeine consumption

PARA-AMINOBENZOIC ACID (PABA)

DEFICIENCY SIGNS   Nervousness, hallucination, depression and digestive upsets

THERAPEUTIC VALUE   Helps prevent the above symptoms and is beneficial to the skin

FOOD SOURCE   Molasses and whole grains

DESTRUCTION   Sulfa drugs

PANTOTHENIC ACID

DEFICIENCY SIGNS   Headache, malaise, nausea, vomiting, leg cramps and flatulence

THERAPEUTIC VALUE   Enables the body to fight infectious diseases and protects against stress, anxiety and depression

FOOD SOURCE   Beans, eggs, fish, vegetables and whole grains

Time has always been spent discussing the need for vitamins, but what about the need for minerals to regain and maintain good health? The following pages cover the minerals the body requires, the problems that result from their deficiencies and the various sources available to insure the alcoholic against mineral loss.

There are three very essential minerals the body requires: calcium, iron and phosphorus. Without adequate amounts of these in the body, severe deficiencies will result and poor health will be inevitable.

CALCIUM

Calcium is the most plentiful mineral in the body. It exists in every living cell. The major part of the mineral is found in the bones and teeth. The heart, muscles and nerve function is dependent upon adequate amounts of calcium. The blood also contains calcium and aids in clotting. The teeth are dependent on calcium for their appearance. Calcium regulates the heart beat and plays an important role in keeping the nerves healthy.

DEFICIENCY SIGNS	Nervousness, muscle weakness, insomnia, irritability, heart palpitation and tooth decay
FOOD SOURCE	Milk, nuts, beans, green vegetables, salmon, sardines (with bones), molasses, Brewer's yeast, cheese and yogurt

IRON

The largest amount of iron is found in the blood. It is essential for energy and a healthy immune system.

DEFICIENCY SIGNS	Fatigue, anemia, paleness, hair loss and dizziness
FOOD SOURCE	Meat, fish, eggs, green vegetables, soy, poultry, whole grains, molasses, raisins, Brewer's yeast and egg yolks

PHOSPHORUS

Phosphorus is responsible for more functions in the body than any other mineral. It is essential to every living cell. It is important to skeletal growth, proper kidney function and heart muscle contraction. Phosphorus, like calcium, is also found in the bones and teeth.

DEFICIENCY SIGNS	Weak muscles, pyorrhea and tooth decay
FOOD SOURCE	Nuts, seeds, bread, eggs, whole grains, garlic, meat, fish, Brewer's yeast, and poultry

POTASSIUM

This mineral is essential for growth, a health nervous system, proper muscle function and regular heartbeat. It works with sodium to maintain water balance in the body.

DEFICIENCY SIGNS	Loss of appetite, muscle weakness, and irritability
FOOD SOURCE	All vegetables, fruits, grains, nuts, Brewer's yeast, fish, beans, poultry, brown rice, potatoes, raisins and garlic

MAGNESIUM

Magnesium is found in the bones, muscles and tissues of the body. It is essential to enzyme activity, aids in maintaining PH balance and helps regulate blood pressure.

DEFICIENCY   Irritability, muscle cramps, twitching,
SIGNS   nervousness, depression, muscle weakness
               and high blood pressure

FOOD SOURCE   Soy beans, nuts, seeds, vegetables, dairy
               products, fish, meat, Brewer's yeast, brown
               rice, whole grains and most fruits

TRACE MINERALS (MICRONUTRIENTS)

Trace minerals are every bit as important to the alcoholic's health as the macronutrients. Although designated amounts have not as yet been determined, it is known that they are needed in lesser quantities and, as with all other minerals, the presence or absence of these denotes the difference between good health and poor health. Trace minerals are necessary to retard certain degenerative processes, for repairing tissues and for metabolic function.

CHROMIUM

Chromium is involved in the metabolism of glucose and enzyme activation. It improves carbohydrate metabolism, the mechanism of the cells and lowers cholesterol and triglyceride levels. Chromium aids in stabilizing the erratic blood sugar seen in alcoholic hypoglycemia. It is effective for sleep disorder in persons with a blood sugar problem. Chromium deficiency has been linked to heart disease.

FOOD SOURCE   Brown rice, cheese, meat, whole grains and
               Brewer's yeast

COBALT

One of the primary problems of cobalt deficiency is progressive nervous system disorder and pernicious anemia.

FOOD SOURCE Wheat germ, eggs, milk, fish, soy beans and Brewer's yeast

COPPER

Small amounts of copper are essential to the alcoholic's health. The specific role that it plays is still undetermined, however one of the most important functions has to do with the red matter of blood (hemoglobin). Copper increases energy, is necessary for healthy skin and nerves.

FOOD SOURCE Beans, molasses, nuts, garlic, raisins, salmon and green leafy vegetables

GERMANIUM

Since germanium enhances cellular oxygenation, it places the immune system in a defensive state. It has also been lauded for its ability as a pain killer.

FOOD SOURCE Garlic, onions, ginseng and shiitake mushroom

IODINE

Iodine manufactures the hormone thyroxin which is indispensable for the thyroid gland. If the thyroid gland is not functioning properly, the metabolic system malfunctions. Over activity, nervousness and irritability are present when the metabolic rate if too rapid. When it is too slow, sluggishness, overweight and laziness occurs. The condition of the hair, skin and nails is also dependent upon an adequate supply of iodine.

FOOD SOURCE   Seafood, kelp, garlic, mushrooms and sea salt

MANGANESE

Manganese is absolutely necessary for the transmission of impulses between the nerves and muscles. It is needed for energy, healthy immune function and protein and fat metabolism.

FOOD SOURCE   Nuts, seeds, wheat germ, whole grains, beans and green leafy vegetables

MOLYBDENUM

This trace mineral is found in the liver. It promotes normal cell function, healthy gums and is only needed in miniscule amounts.

FOOD SOURCE   Beans, whole grains and green leafy vegetables

SELENIUM

Tissue elasticity is preserved when adequate amounts of selenium are present. Vitamin E and selenium work synergistically. Together, they can slow down the signs of aging considerably. Selenium protects the immune system from free radicals and aids in the production of antibodies.

FOOD SOURCE   Brewer's yeast, wheat germ, onion, garlic, chicken, whole grains, meat, brown rice and tomatoes

SILICON

Silicon is necessary for healthy hair, skin and nails. It plays a vital role in maintaining a healthy heart.

FOOD SOURCE   Brown rice, green bell peppers, whole grains
and green leafy vegetables

SULFUR

The skin, bones and muscles of the body contain sulfur. Sulfur contributes to the process of metabolizing fat and of significance to alcoholics as it stimulates bile secretions in the liver, protecting it from toxicity.

FOOD SOURCE   Red peppers and eggs contain the highest
content. Other foods are onions, garlic,
brussel sprouts, broccoli, beans and cabbage

VANADIUM

Vanadium is essential for cellular metabolism. It promotes cardiovascular and reproductive health. It plays a role in growth and formation of bones and teeth.

FOOD SOURCE   Fish, meat and whole grains

ZINC

Zinc promotes a healthy immune system, enhances the healing process, is necessary for hair growth and glowing skin. It is essential for prostate gland and reproductive organ functions.

FOOD SOURCE   Beans, nuts, seafood, poultry, meat, Brewer's
yeast, whole grains, sardines and seeds

Having read this chapter on vitamins and minerals, their requirements for various organs, glands and body parts, it is plain to see the vital role they play in regaining and maintaining the integrity of the cellular environment of the malnourished alcoholic.

While reading the suggested weekly menu, you may have viewed it as somewhat repetitious. Soup, vegetables and salad, along with whole grains, meat or fish was mentioned daily. However, while looking to the food source for the nutrient value of foods, it is easy to see why the previous menus, although simplistic in design, offer a power-house program.

There is a veritable garden for health out there and is everyone's for the taking. Over the years, many lives have been transformed through a sound nutritional program and the application of same. When the body, mind and emotion are nourished, the alcoholic no longer just walks through life, but lives it.

HISTORICAL USES OF HERBS

Due to the disease of alcoholism, the body experiences a tremendous amount of abuse, but it can receive considerable support through the use of herbs. They perform many healing functions in the body and have been used for centuries for their medicinal properties.

Although the list of herbs that follow have proved highly beneficial to health and well-being, it is not the intent of the author to diagnose or prescribe, but to offer health information. In the event you use this information without your doctor's approval, you are then prescribing for yourself, which is your constitutional right.

HERB	USES
ALFALFA	Anemia, blood purifier, digestive disorders, energy and hypoglycemia

PAULINE GRAY

ANGELICA	Tonic for mind and body. Noted for its help with spleen disorders
ASTRAGALUS	Enhances immune response, reduces edema, increases metabolism and energy
ALOE VERA	Burns, constipation, liver, wounds and digestive disorders
BARBERRY	Blood purifier, liver and gallbladder (promotes bile secretion).
BEE POLLEN	Allergies, energy and hypoglycemia
BLACK COHOSH	Natural supplier of estrogen, liver, blood purifier, circulation, lowers blood pressure and cholesterol, hot flashes, kidneys and menstrual cramps
BLACK WALNUT	Cleanses the body of parasites, tape worms and ring worm
BLADDERWRACK	Enhances kidney function and increases thyroid activity
BLESSED THISTLE	Heals the liver, increases and enriches Mother's milk, purifies the blood, digestive disorders and menstrual cramps
BLUE COHOSH	Cramps, nervous disorders, blood purifier and elevates blood pressure

SOBER FOR THE HEALTH OF IT

BUCHU	Urinary disorders, edema, prostate, hypolgycemia and gas
BUCKTHORN	Constipation, gall stones and liver
BURDOCK	Blood purifier, arthritic joints, energy, nervous disorders, skin problems, edema, stimulates the immune system and restores liver and gallbladder function
BUTCHERS BROOM	Kidneys, liver, leg cramps and gout
CAMOMILE	Cleanser for drug use, gas, improves appetite, digestive disorders, insomnia, nervousness and parasites
CASCARA SAGRADA	Used mainly for liver disorders, gall stones, stomach, pancreas, spleen and constipation
CATNIP	Diarrhea, hypoglycemia, insomnia, nervousness, stress and edema
CAYENNE	One of natures greatest herbs. It stops internal bleeding, helps regulate blood pressure, improves circulation, cleans out bronchial tubes when used with ginger, aids digestion, stimulates the heart, increases energy, good for the kidneys, lungs, liver, spleen, pancreas, yeast infections and hemorrhoids

CHICKWEED	Gastrointestinal disorders, appetite suppressant, reduces mucous build-up in the respiratory tract
COMFREY	Anemia, blood purifier, digestive disorders, lungs, kidneys and sinus congestion
CORNSILK	Uterine disorders and painful urination due to prostate gland problems. Water retention, liver and constipation
COUCH GRASS	Water retention, liver and constipation
DAMIANA	(Female herb) relieving hot flashes and increasing libido
DANDELION	Anemia, blood builder, blood purifier, liver cleanser, gall bladder, kidneys, hypoglycemia, pancreas, stomach and spleen
DONG QUAI	(Female herb) vaginal dryness, hot flashes, energy, menstrual cramps, hypoglycemia and menopause. Not to be taken during pregnancy
ECHINACEA	Blood purifier, immune system and lymph glands
FENNEL	Appetite normalizer, gas, liver, digestive disorders, spleen and kidneys

FENUGREEK	Digestive disorders, sinus congestion and migraine headaches
GARLIC	A natural antibiotic similar to penicillin. Used for detoxification, high blood pressure, gas, liver, digestive disorders, parasites, prostate gland, sinusitis and yeast infections
GINGER	Antacid, spastic colon, gas, nausea and digestive disorders
GINKO BILOBA	Memory loss, depression, circulation, heart and kidneys
GINSENG	Impotence, drug withdrawal, asthma, endurance, prostate gland and vitality
GOLDEN SEAL	Antibiotic, hypoglycemia, liver, spleen, pancreas, stomach, digestion, prostate gland, circulation, sinus congestion and vaginal disorders
GOTU KOLA	Memory loss, nervousness, fatigue, depression, insomnia, liver and heart function
HAWTHORN	Adrenal glands, hypoglycemia, energy, blood pressure (high or low), water retention and heart disease

HOPS	Decreases the desire for alcohol, insomnia, liver, nervousness and night sweats
HOREHOUND	Coughs, colds, nasal and chest congestion
HORSETAIL	Body odor, hair, skin, nails edema and nervousness
HYSSOP	Mucous, blood pressure, digestive disorders, liver, night sweats and sore throat
IRISH MOSS	Regulation of thyroid gland (high iodine content)
JUNIPER	Hypoglycemia, adrenal glands, kidneys, sinusitis and edema
KELP	Hypoglycemia, adrenal glands, obesity, pituitary gland and thyroid
LICORICE ROOT	Drug withdrawal, hypoglycemia, energy, pancreas, nausea, mild laxative
LOBELIA	Powerful relaxant, cough suppressant, nervousness, liver and muscle spasm
MANDRAKE	Liver, gall bladder and constipation
MARSHMALLOW	Hypoglycemia, bladder, kidneys, mucous membranes, nervousness and urinary disorders

MILKWEED	Gastrointestinal tract, gall bladder and kidneys
MULLEIN	Asthma, bronchitis, diarrhea, pain, swollen glands and sinus congestion
MYRRH	Hypoglycemia, colitis, digestive disorders, nervousness, thrush and hypothyroidism
NETTLE	Kidney stones and urinary problems
OATSTRAW	Arthritis, hair, nails, kidneys, liver and nervousness
PARSLEY	Arthritis, bad breath, kidneys, liver, edema, gas and stomach
PAU D'ARCO	Blood purifier, yeast infection, liver disease and all infections in general
PASSION FLOWER	Alcoholism, headaches, nervousness and insomnia
PEPPERMINT	Digestive disorders, nervousness, appetite stimulant, gas, nausea and liver
POKE WEED	Inflammation, liver, lymph glands and thyroid
PUMPKIN SEED	Prostate gland, stomach and nausea
RED CLOVER	Relaxant, acne and blood purifier

RED RASPBERRY	Diarrhea, female disorders, flu, nausea and canker sores
ROSE HIPS	Infections, colds and stress
SAFFLOWER	Hypoglycemia, muscle cramps, gout, fatigue, liver and edema
SAGE	Gastrointestinal tract, mouth sores, nervousness and night sweats
SARSAPARILLA	Blood purifier, impotence, liver, stress, all skin disorders, regulation of male and female hormones
SAW PALMETTO	Alcoholism, swollen glands and regulation of hormones
SKULLCAP	Alcoholism, relaxant, insomnia, hypoglycemia and nervousness
SLIPPERY ELM	Digestion, diarrhea, sore throat, stomach and urinary tract
SPEARMINT	Same properties as peppermint, but milder
ST. JOHNS WORT	Depression, nervousness and edema
SUMA	Immune system, stress and fatigue
THYME	Mucous build-up, digestive disorders, kidney stone prevention and headache

UVA URSI	Urinary tract infections and edema
VALERIAN	Alcoholism, insomnia, nervousness and anxiety
WHITE OAK BARK	Yeast infections, canker sores, hemorrhoids, varicose veins and thrush
WOOD BETONY	Headaches, relaxant for nervous disorders
YARROW	Bladder, blood purifier, colds, congestion, diarrhea, insomnia, skin problems and sore throat
YELLOW DOCK	Blood purifier, liver, energy, skin problems and anemia
YERBAMATE	Blood purifier, nervousness and said to retard aging
YUCCA	Arthritis, rheumatism, gout and blood purifier

The aforementioned herbs can be taken as a tea. However, some of the herbs are not particularly palatable, but can be used effectively in the form of capsules.

Every alcoholic who is sincerely striving for health and vitality will reach his/her full potential by listening to his/her body.

A new way of life can be discovered through proper diet, vitamins, minerals and herbs.

12

CAN ALCOHOLISM BE PREVENTED

Alcoholism, a common prob-
lem in many households, is considered incurable. This is
connected with the failure of cells, in the body, to function
normally. Good nutrition assures us that the cells will regenerate faster and work longer, if they are furnished with the proper
fuel. Can alcoholism be cured? Perhaps not, due to massive cellular damage. The next question then should be, can alcoholism be prevented?

Researchers and various health agencies realize the importance of coming up with definitive answers in coping with the
disease of alcoholism. The causative factors of psychological
abnormalities are always under speculation. One cannot deny
that it is partly psychological, but also physical. Regardless of
the attention, the researchers still aren't clear as to what actually
causes this disease.

SOBER FOR THE HEALTH OF IT

There is evidence that alcoholism can be hereditary and/or caused by biochemical imbalance. Still there are those who see this disease, not as a cellular environment problem, but one precipitated by learned behavior patterns.

In her practice, the author has made a case for qualitative as well as quantitative nutritional therapy. Progress has been made in other areas of disease in respect to causative factors, but this is not the case with the disease of alcoholism. Nutritional treatment has not been emphasized. Over the years, too many health care providers have stated, "The alcoholic can only deal with one problem at a time. It's difficult enough staying sober without having to make choices about which food they should or should not eat." There are some excellent theories in the area of nutrition/alcoholism that are worth exploration by the medical profession namely: hypoglycemia, allergies and chemical imbalance. It may prove pertinent in the area of prevention. Abstaining from alcohol does not necessarily mean a person is well, but being sober for the health of it makes all the difference to the mental, physical and emotional well-being of the alcoholic.

The following tables represent the major symptoms experienced by 74 alcoholics (sobriety ranging from 4 weeks to 18 months).

MAJOR SYMPTOMS EXPERIENCED BY 74 RECOVERING ALCOHOLICS

SYMPTOMS	PERCENT OF CLIENTS REPORTING SYMPTOMS
PSYCHIATRIC	
ANXIETY	80

DEPRESSION 72

IRRITABILITY 67

FORGETFULNESS/CONFUSION 48

RESTLESSNESS 47

LACK OF CONCENTRATION 41

ANTISOCIAL BEHAVIOR 18

INSOMNIA 15

SUICIDAL TENDENCY 5

SOMATIC

FATIGUE 82

TACHYCARDIA 46

CHRONIC 45
INDIGESTION/BLOATING

JOINT PAINS 33

EXCESSIVE SWEATING 29

COLD HANDS/FEET 28

NEUROLOGIC

MUSCLE PAIN/BACKACHE 92

MUSCULAR TWITCHING/CRAMPS 81

TREMOR (INWARD/OUTWARD)	66
DIZZINESS	64
HEADACHES	48
· NUMBNESS	33

The following table shows the improvements experienced by two experimental groups. A close watch was kept on the diet and nutritional supplementation of Group 1. The second group was given a sound diet to follow, but without food supplementation. This experiment took place over a ten week period.

SYMPTOM	GROUP I (37 CLIENTS)	GROUP 2 (37 CLIENTS)
PSYCHIATRIC		
ANXIETY	2	33
DEPRESSION	14	36
IRRITABILITY	17	32
FORGETFULNESS/CONFUSION	3	13
RESTLESSNESS	9	17
LACK OF CONCENTRATION	8	19
ANTISOCIAL BEHAVIOR	19	31
INSOMNIA	6	34

SUICIDAL TENDENCY	I	3

SOMATIC

FATIGUE	19	34
TACHYCARDIA	7	23
CHRONIC INDIGESTION/BLOATING	4	29
JOINT PAINS	8	17
EXCESSIVE SWEATING	18	31
COLD HANDS/FEET	3	26

NEUROLOGIC

MUSCLE PAIN/BACKACHE	4	20
MUSCULAR TWITCHING/CRAMPS	8	29
TREMOR (INWARD/OUTWARD)	14	23
DIZZINESS	16	37
HEADACHES	7	35
NUMBNESS	13	21

Group 1 also received herbs to initiate cleansing of the bowel, liver, pancreas and digestive system. They were also placed on a variety of herbs to enhance the body's healing power. They did considerably well in a short time and all were pleased and greatly surprised by the marked improvement in their health.

Prevention of this disease may be possible, but education

must begin at an early age. We all have a body, and yet, few know how it functions. How does the food we eat and beverages we drink affect it? If we learned at an early age that we were predisposed to a variety of illnesses, we would have the ammunition to enable us to make conscious decisions regarding our state of health. It would be a case of "Let the buyer beware."

We live in a society that promotes the concept that love, sex, and all fun times go hand-in-hand with drinking alcohol. Television commercials show the drinking of alcohol to be desirable and attractive. They never show the person losing their family, job, home and self-respect. We are not shown the slow case of suicide that goes on within the body of the alcoholic. However, the nightly news does show the tragedies involved due to an intoxicated driver behind the wheel of a car.

Cigarette commercials have been banned because smoking them has proved hazardous to our health. Commercials endorsing a product that is every bit as deadly as tobacco, namely alcohol, should also be removed since our youth is so impressionable.

When all is said and done, "We are the product of what we eat, drink and think."

13

SUMMARY

THE NUMBER OF PEOPLE afflicted
with the disease of alcoholism is overwhelming. It has even
found its' way into our grammar school system. Reported cases
have covered a wide age range from 9 years and up. Alcohol
abuse is shattering lives. Teenagers are being devastated by violence and incarceration. The earlier in life these youths begin
to drink alcohol, the more likely they are to experiment with
a variety of drugs. This same type of experimentation causes
what is known as dual addiction.

The facts surrounding pre-teen and teenage alcoholism is
alarming. Dr. Gordis, director of NIAAA states, "Our nation
can no longer ignore alcohol use in children. Scientific evidence
shows that the earlier children begin drinking, the more likely
they are to develop serious alcohol problems in their lifetime."

Although marijuana and cocaine are presenting a problem

among the youth in the United States, alcoholism is still the number one addiction. It appears that drinking is more socially acceptable than the use of the aforementioned drugs. Alcohol abuse is causing fatal car accidents, broken homes, suicide and giving way to a nation of seriously ill people.

Alcohol consumption is the leading cause of injury and death among America's youth.

Alcoholism effects more than the abuser. It takes its' toll on their families, society and has economic consequences, as well.

The National Institute on Alcohol Abuse and Alcoholism states, "In purely economic terms, alcohol abuse and alcoholism cost an estimated $184.6 billion per year. In human terms, the costs are incalculable."

Alcohol and women has become a significant issue in the past two decades. Females have narrowed the gap between themselves and their male counterpart. Although both sexes will experience physical and psychological harm due to their increased alcohol consumption, there are problems special to women. One of the most profound tragedies results when pregnant women abuse alcohol. The impact on the unborn child can be devastating. Multiple abnormalities can occur due to Fetal Alcohol Syndrome. Central nervous system dysfunction, altered prenatal growth and mental retardation, are just a few of the deleterious effects on the unborn child. Intervention is of the utmost importance since two lives are at risk.

Of all the alcoholics in the United States, the mentally ill are the most visible. Facilities are filled to capacity with these dually disabled people and once they are stabilized, they are discharged. They are homeless, unable to cope in the community and left to wander the streets aimlessly. The difficulty in treating them comes from the opposing approaches taken by the mental health professionals and the substance abuse counselors.

Behavior is due, in part, to metabolic disorder. Proper diet, or lack thereof, influences the endocrine glands. Abnormal biochemical profiles have been seen in individuals with psychological disorders as well as alcoholics.

The American Medical Association and the director of the Substance Abuse and Mental Health Services Administration claim, "We have an epidemic of alcohol abuse among the elderly."

Since aging, for some, is a time of diminished physical and psychological capacity, the symptoms of alcoholism may go undetected for a considerable period of time. In a younger individual cognitive decline, recurrent accidents and estrangement from family would be linked to chronic alcoholism. However, any or all of the above may be experienced by the elderly.

The elderly who are on medication are adversely effected by alcohol. They may experience further confusion and even physical toxicity. Alcohol/medication interaction has been known to be extremely dangerous or fatal. Physicians and family members need to monitor the elderly person's prescription and over-the-counter medications. Alcohol mixed with medication can have devastating consequences.

Hospitalization is necessary when the alcoholic is in a life or death situation, but even those institutions that specialize in alcohol rehabilitation do not emphasize proper diet. Eating from the four basic food groups does not necessarily bring about good health and well-being. Most hospital dieticians put together "balanced diets." The alcoholic patient is then allowed to eat any amount of sugar laden foods and drink coffee the major part of the day. This is a destructive pattern since it has been established that many alcoholics are hypoglycemic and require a specialized diet. Alcoholics body's have been stressed to the limit and require a program that will meet their individual biochemical needs to create a balance within the organism.

The excessive ingestion of alcohol associated with alcoholism causes extreme, multiple nutrient deficiencies. Once intervention takes place it is essential to have the alcoholic begin a whole foods approach to eating. Along with eating well, meaningful amounts of food supplements should be taken to encourage cellular renewal and reduce the toxic effects associated with the disease of alcoholism. Amelioration of the symptoms of alcohol withdrawal and cravings are evident.

Reducing toxicity is important to the welfare of the alcoholic. Many of the effects experienced by the alcoholic are due, not only to the alcohol, but to the drugs administered by the physician and the nutritional deficiencies as well. Nutritional supplementation for alcoholics can have a prophylactic effect. Vitamins A, C and E, taken in conjunction with zinc and selenium work on building the body's immune system. In addition, the nutritional approach may possibly protect the liver from the ravages due to excessive alcohol.

The author's personal studies were performed on three groups of alcoholics. It was noted that alcohol cravings were associated with diets high in refined carbohydrates. The second group was placed on a diet high in raw foods. This prompted temporary avoidance of alcohol. The chronic alcoholics who ate a whole foods diet, accompanied by food supplements, did far better with long term abstaining from alcohol. Diets consisting solely of refined carbohydrates caused the alcoholic to slide back, and at times, even increase alcohol intake.

Allergies to specific foods (corn, wheat and yeast) may also cause alcohol cravings. These are three of the known offenders. Scientific evidence is lacking regarding food sensitivity. Being on a nutritionally well-balanced diet with adequate food supplementation suggests metabolic controls.

Nutritional deficiencies come, for the most part, from ethanol toxicity, the alcoholic experiences gastrointestinal problems, weight loss and vomiting. An electrolyte imbalance becomes apparent and specific nutrient deficiencies exist including thiamine (B1), folic acid, calcium, magnesium and the fat soluble vitamins (A, D, E).

Failure of protein synthesis and amino acid imbalance is prominent among alcoholics with liver disease. Controlled vitamin A supplementation should be taken along with other vitamins especially during detoxification to resolve hypovitaminosis. Liver toxicity is enhanced by chronic alcohol consumption even in the early stages of involvement. Avitaminosis has been known to cause night blindness and cirrhosis in alcoholics.

Supplementing with B complex is crucial. Alcoholics experience all of the classic symptoms of thiamine, pyridoxine, B12 and folic acid deficiencies. This is due to inadequate intake and the inability to absorb foods. Thirty seven clients were put on 100mg. of B complex daily along with a whole foods diet and claimed a decrease in their craving for alcohol.

Alcoholics with gastrointestinal malabsorption have significantly low folate levels. With supplementation and abstinence the folate levels increase.

Chronic ingestion of the ethanol in alcohol reduces the B3 levels causing irritability and restlessness. Supplementation appears to be one effective means of treating the alcoholic with delirium tremens. Chronic alcoholics with liver disease show a B3 deficiency.

Of the seventy four clients observed by the author, all were deficient in riboflavin.

Thiamine deficiency has been known to be responsible for the neurological condition of Wernick's syndrome.

All alcoholics in this study group were deficient in B1, B2, B6, B12 and folic acid. This would account for the neurological disorders experienced.

Since ethanol produces toxicity in the alcoholic liver, ascorbic acid (vitamin C) may have a protective effect against alcohol toxicity when taken in ample amounts.

Of the seventy four clients tested, all had low calcium magnesium levels. Intracellular depletion is due to excessive urination. Deficiency of magnesium in chronic alcoholics can cause cardiovascular disease.

Alcohol abuse is associated with zinc deficiency. Those clients with zinc deficiency took 50mg. daily for a six week period and demonstrated a heightened degree of taste and smell.

Lglutamine has been known to diminish the craving for alcohol and supplies the brain with energy. Out of the thirty seven clients who took Lglutamine, thirty four had decreased anxiety and their sleep improved.

Over the years, various modalities have attempted to deal with the alcoholics illness, however, none has proven quite as successful as the nutritional approach to the treatment of alcoholism. Psychoanalysis has its' place, but does nothing to correct nutrient deficiencies in patients. While the psycho-pharmacologic aspect may appeal to some (to treat acute symptoms) this approach only complicates the already complex situation. The drugs side effects mimic the very symptoms being experienced by the recovering alcoholic during their withdrawal period. This causes great confusion.

Support groups for alcoholics and non- alcoholics are beneficial. They are educational, informative and enable an individual to restructure their life. A successful support group, known the world over, is Alcoholics Anonymous. One of its' more recognized co-founders was a gentleman by the name of Bill Wilson. He found out, early in his sobriety, that good foods and nutritional supplementation gave aid to the alcoholic. Through biochemical rebalancing, via proper nutrition, the physical, mental and emotional problems will resolve themselves as the body heals. Once again, or perhaps for the first time, optimal health will be experienced.

The road back requires patience, understanding and perseverance. It means living life—"One Day At A Time."

APPENDIX A

THE FOLLOWING IS A transcript of a presentation given by the author at a community meeting February 28, 2005. It was given in response to the topic "Not in MY Neighborhood." It is included in this book to help the reader realize the vulnerability of all of us and to reach out to the community for better understanding.

The last time I spoke to you, I talked about the need for change in the treatment programs for the hospitalized alcoholic. Today, I would like to speak on a more personal note. The story you are about to hear is not limited to those of us in this room, but concerns all people in general. It's about people's experiences whether they be good, bad or indifferent. It speaks to the body, mind and spirit. It addresses fear, doubt, hate and acceptance. This story is about love, sharing and the ability to open our minds and heart to *all* beings. It's about acceptance.

Meetings, similar to this, have been given in various communities. It's a time of coming together to create some type of peace and a better understanding of, not only our neighbor, but ourselves.

I want you to take the next few minutes to think about the one person or thing that is troubling you the most. Nothing, you say? Come on, let's be honest. Is it the winter months you couldn't wait for when the heat wave hit? Is it your husband/wife's drinking? Perhaps it's your wife's unending questions about why you were late for diner and how you spend your idle time that causes you grief. None of these problems? Very unlikely, but I'll move on. How about the dessert you gave into which threw you off your diet, or the upsetment on the job which caused you to go back to smoking. Didn't get to it yet? Well, I'm sure you'll think of something.

Let's review a few of these situations. You may think I'm going to get a little crazy with my explanations, but bear with me on this one. Be grateful for this time for it's going to be your chance to experience life. It's the reason you drew your first breath. I heard what you just thought. I drew my first breath to put up with this person's drinking problem, to listen to her nagging, to walk around forty pounds overweight? We've all been given a lesson plan and perhaps for some it's to learn patience, for another humility and for most of us, the ability to be open to change and new ideas. For now, let's attempt to erase all time. Try to open your minds and take in as much of the following as is possible. You have the ability to change *your* environment.

The word 'your' is emphasized because I mean exactly that. The need for change is within you. In doing so, changes in everything else around you will happen systematically.

Let's go back to the drawing board, a time before your birth. For now, just for the sake of making a point, let's call it "Messages From The Other Side." Close your eyes and visualize a roll of theatre tickets with numbers ranging from one through nine. For every tenth person, the numbers repeat themselves.

Let's say that all those who drew the #1 (a powerful number indeed) were born to an alcoholic parent and then, to complicate matters, married into alcoholism or became alcoholics themselves. The #2 people came forward to lead impoverished lives, while the #3 went on to fame and fortune, never to experience a private life and seldom peace. The #4's married several times and were never truly happy in any marriage. If affordable, these people wound up in therapy. Number 5 people will be the angry ones wandering through life domineering and manipulating as many lives as time permits. Those who drew #6 were born to the religious life and were to wrestle, from time to time, with their conviction, perhaps encountering moments of weakness. Number 7, poor souls, always trying to get something for nothing. Number 8, what could be left? You got it. You were born a minority and to this very day there are those among us who would say, "Please step to the rear of the bus." "Thank goodness," say those with the number nine, "all the garbage has been handed out. It's time for the good life." Sorry #9, you got it all. You'll be born into the alcoholic household and experience child abuse (be it verbal or physical). Perhaps your parents are clean, but you take to drugs and/or alcohol. Due to this lifestyle, material things won't be plentiful for most.

However, you were born with good looks and a style all your own. You go on to meet someone who will take you out of your impoverished state. You too have a tendency toward being arrogant with those less fortunate than yourself, forgetting from whence you came. Perhaps you'll get into a jam or two. Maybe it will be the speeding ticket or the DWI you fight in court, after all, you only had four drinks. Let's not forget that #9's are part of the minority and for this go round, you drew the ticket labeled 'gay man,' 'lesbian woman.' PLEASE STEP TO THE REAR OF THE BUS.

What is this session all about? It's about coming to the realization that we are all vulnerable to life and what it has to offer. We are all made of cells, and are just a cellular extension of each other. Each breath I exhale, someone will inhale and visa versa. Since the time of your birth, your true nature was joyful, loving, peaceful and giving—free from sadness, fear, doubt and hate. Somewhere along the way, we got side tracked.

Over the years, an insidious disease has developed within some of you. The numbers continue to grow at an alarming rate. Tonight, I hope, messages from the other side has given each of you the opportunity to raise your level of consciousness to some degree.

We all know one of the words that makes us feel uncomfortable and degraded. That word is alcoholic. Each of us in this room needs to learn as much as we possibly can about alcoholism. This disease debilitates the afflicted on all cellular levels.

I do hope this hour will give each of you the opportunity to search inside yourself. Some people have become frightened and embittered toward the alcoholic, but we need to see that the disease frightens the alcoholic as well. They also become bitter toward life and all that it has to offer.

Seeds of hate are often planted in the subconscious mind and nurtured through negative actions. This chokes out a positive lifestyle. Learning to remove the garbage from our minds and replacing it with positive thoughts will help us change mentally, physically and emotionally. Some of us have built a house of nothing but stone walls. Through experience, we can add windows to let in the light of day, and a door to set us free.

Alcoholism has given all those involved sorrow, anguish and pain. We have a long row to hoe. Healing this country of this disease is easier said than done.

We are the sum total of all our parts and should be treated thusly. You cannot separate body, mind and emotion. Setting up centers that would address the entire being are necessary. Education is crucial. Abstaining from alcohol, for the most part, is being dry. Mental clarity, emotional stability and an overall sense of well-being adds up to being SOBER FOR THE HEALTH OF IT.

Editor's Note: Messages from The Other Side has been delivered on numerous occasions, has been well received by those in attendance and above all, makes its' point.

BIBLIOGRAPHY

Adleman, Steve, M.D., Drugs and Medication, 2000

Alagna, Madelena, The Dangers of Binge Drinking. The Rosen Publishing Group Inc. 2001

Alcoholics Anonymous, Revised Edition, 16th Printing, 1974

Alcohol Induced Deaths, Alcohol Statistics 2002

Alcohol, Violence and Crime, National Violence Against Women Survey, 1993

American Academy of Child and Adolescent Psychiatry, 1997

American Journal of Public Health, COA's Survey, JN 2000

Archives of General Psychiatry, Volume 56, 1999

Alanon Family Group Headquarters, Inc., Hope for Children of Alcoholics: Alateen, 5th Printing, 1980

Blum A.W., et.al., Department of Psychiatry Harborview Medical Center, 2000

Brooks, Courtenay, Alcohol Consumption and Cardiac Death, American Family Physicians, March 2000

SOBER FOR THE HEALTH OF IT

Brower, Kirk, Alcohols Effects on Sleep in Alcoholics, 2001

Berggren, U, et.al., Extremely Long Recovery Time, Amedeo Internet Services, 2002

Columbia Center of Addiction and Substance Abuse, Elderly Americans and Alcohol, July 1998

Donahue, Richard P. et.al., Journal of the American Medical Association 255:2311-2314, May 1986

Dorlands Illustrated Medical Dictionary, March 2000

Doyle, Roger, Deaths Due to Alcohol, Scientific American, 1996

Ernest Gallo Clinic and Research Center, Alcohol and the Brain, Neurology Dept. April 2002

Enoch Gordis M.D., Teens and Alcohol Don't Mix, April 2001

Fletcher, Anne M., Sober for Good, Houghton Mifflin and Company, 2001

Garbutt, J.C., M.D., Pharmacological Treatment for Alcoholism, Bowles Center for Alcohol Studies, 2002

Greenhaven Press, Inc. Drunk Driving, 2001

Harwood, et.al., Economic Costs of Alcohol Abuse in the U.S., 2000

Hazeldon Foundation, 12 Step Wisdom at Work: Transforming Your Life and Your Organization, 2001

Holder, Jay, D.C., University of Miami School of Medicine, The Brain Reward Cascade, 1993

Huffman, Grace, American Family Physicians, November 1999

Institute of Pharmacology and Psychiatry, Rome, Italy, 2000

Ketcham, Katherine, Beyond the Influence: Understanding and Defeating Alcoholism, Bantam Books, 2000

Kokin, Morris, Women Married to Alcoholics, William Morrow & Co., Inc. 1989

Mark, Tami L., Ph.D., Physicians Perceptions and Use of Alcoholism Medications, The MEDSTAT Group, 2002

Munro, Robin, M.D., Yoga Biomedical Trust: Alternative Medicine Handbook, the Burton Group, 1993

Nakken, Craig, *Reclaim Your Family from Addiction*, Hazeldon, 2000

National Institute of Drug Abuse and Health, Alcohol and Pregnancy, Health Survey, 1992

National Institute of Health, FAS, JN 2001

NIAAA, Cumulative Effects of Alcohol, 1996

National Highway Traffic Safety Administration, Alcohol Highway Safety, 1998

NIH, Research Insights into Alcoholism and Alcohol Abuse, News Advisory, Special Report, NV 2000

Okoro Cyprian, M.D., Repeat Inpatient Rehabilitation, STEER, 2001

Peele Stanton, Ph.D., Alcoholism and the Elderly, American Medical Association, July 1998

Schaefer, Dick, Choices & Consequences: What To Do When a Teenager Uses Alcohol/Drugs, 1987

Sciacca, Kathleen, New Directions for Mental Health Services, 1991

Secretary of Health and Human Services, Alcohol and Health Report to Congress, June 2000

Swanson, Christine, M.D., Heavy Drinking Associated with Higher Risk of Breast Cancer, Epiden, 1997

Summers, Suzanne, *Wednesdays' Child*, Putnam/Healing Vision Publishing, 1992

The Indiana Prevention Resource Center, Indiana University, Survey August 2001

Tsukamoto, H., LuSc., Current Concepts of Pathogenesis of Alcoholic Liver Injury, 2001

ABOUT THE AUTHOR

Aᴌᴛʜᴏᴜɢʜ ɪɴ ʜᴇʀ sᴇᴠᴇɴᴛɪᴇs, Pauline Gray is a radiant woman who seems to pulsate with great energy.

Her introduction to a holistic modality began in 1965 when she enrolled in a series of Hatha Yoga classes with Richard Hittleman. This encounter with wellness caused her interest to grow in leaps and bounds.

From 1972 until her retirement in April 2000, she practiced holistically. During those twenty eight years, she received her Ph.D. in nutrition. She later became certified in nutritional consulting from the American Association of Nutritional Consultants. She studied herbology with Dr. John Christopher, became a certified and registered foot reflexologist (practicing the original Ingham method). Gray studied iridology with the man who pioneered it in the U.S.—Dr. Bernard Jensen and

PAULINE GRAY

received her D. Sc. Degree in Pastoral Psychology.

All who have known Dr. Gray agree, "She is a true caregiver in every sense of the word, and her talent and ambition seems limitless."

In 1985 Pauline received a nutritional science award in recognition of Distinguished Achievement in Natural Nutrition.

She designed and authored a Comprehensive Iridology/ Herbology course which was approved in 1992 by the New York State Nurses Association for continuing credits. This course was taught to nurses and chiropractors in the states of Florida, Georgia and New York.

December 1993 Gray received her license from the Pastoral Care Licensing Commission.

In late 1994 Pauline was given the Sister Mary Thomas award in recognition of the many hours donated to the church as a pastoral counselor for the lay community and clergy.

Throughout the years, she has worked diligently and been a role model for her belief, "Neither science nor adjunct natural therapies says it all. We each need to be forthright about our limitations. It's time we emerged from our respective corners to work in tandem towards wholeness."

Member—American Association of Nutritional Consultants
International Women's Writing Guild

ISBN 142512121-7